PENGUIN BOOKS

48 HOURS TO A HEALTHIER LIFE

Suzi Grant worked as a radio and TV journalist and presenter for over twenty years. Having had enough of such a stressful life, she trained as a nutritional therapist and now runs practices in London and Brighton. She is also a health journalist and writes for magazines, runs workshops and appears regularly on radio and TV.

48 Hours to a Healthier Life is her first book. You can find more information on Suzi Grant on her website: www.benatural.co.uk

48
Hours to a Healthier Life

SUZI GRANT

PENGUIN BOOKS

PENGUIN BOOKS

Published by the Penguin Group
Penguin Books Ltd, 80 Strand, London WC2R ORL, England
Penguin Putnam Inc., 375 Hudson Street, New York, New York 10014, USA
Penguin Books Australia Ltd, 250 Camberwell Road,
Camberwell, Victoria 3124, Australia
Penguin Books Canada Ltd, 10 Alcorn Avenue, Toronto, Ontario, Canada M4V 3B2
Penguin Books India (P) Ltd, 11 Community Centre,
Panchsheel Park, New Delhi – 110 017, India
Penguin Books (NZ) Ltd, Cnr Rosedale and Airborne Roads,
Albany, Auckland, New Zealand
Penguin Books (South Africa) (Pty) Ltd, 24 Sturdee Avenue,
Rosebank 2196, South Africa

Penguin Books Ltd, Registered Offices: 80 Strand, London WC2R ORL, England

www.penguin.com

First published 2003
8

Set in Monotype Fournier
Typeset by Rowland Phototypesetting Ltd, Bury St Edmunds, Suffolk
Printed in England by Clays Ltd, St Ives plc

Contents

Warning   vii
Foreword   ix
Introduction   xi

1. The Philosophy: Natural Nutrition   1
2. Preparing for Your Weekend   12
3. **H** for H$_2$O: Water   30
4. **E** for Eliminating the Challenging Foods   39
5. **A** for Alternatives   57
6. **L** for Lymph   74
7. **T** for Tackling Toxins   85
8. **H** for Hydrotherapy   103
9. **I** for Immunity and Immune Response   111
10. **E** for Exercise   121
11. **R** for Rhythms   135
12. **L** for Liver   146
13. **I** for Integration   156
14. **F** for Fats: The Essential Ones   166
15. **E** for Exit Routes   177

16. The Plan!   189
17. Recipe Suggestions   213
18. How to Carry on in the Real World   245

Acknowledgements   257
Further Reading and Information   258

Warning

If you are pregnant, planning to become pregnant, breastfeeding, on any form of medication, chronically ill, likely to suffer an allergic reaction, very young or very old, please seek professional advice before trying any treatment, herb, essential oil, food or beverage recommended in this book!

Foreword

In my thirties, I was a chain-smoking, hard-drinking TV journalist. When my mother died of a sudden heart attack, at the age of sixty-one, I started asking questions. We come from a long line of people blessed by longevity – at least on the female side of the family. But my – previously healthy – mother took little or no exercise, started smoking at the age of sixty, was very overweight and didn't care what she ate – as long as it tasted good! She was unfit, unhappy and uninspired.

It was my wake-up call and, like anyone else reading this who has lost a loved one in the prime of his or her life, I decided to take more control of my health. Not just for the sake of my body, but for the sake of my mental and emotional states as well, so I could lead a happier life than my mother led at the end.

My path of learning led me to train as a Nutritional Therapist. Originally I didn't intend to treat people – I just wanted the knowledge to become a more credible health writer. But the health benefits I experienced, as can anyone else prepared to make a few simple changes to their lifestyle and diet, proved to be so dramatic and swift that I just had to continue spreading the word!

I don't live on the top of a mountain, don't meditate every morning at 6 a.m. and don't avoid alcohol as if it were produced by the devil himself. Nor do any of my patients. But I do look after my physical and mental health by taking 'time out' to relax, exercising regularly, eating 'life-giving' foods and indulging in the 'bad stuff' only in moderation.

I have learned and experienced what Eastern mystics have known for thousands of years. In the short term, making very simple changes to lifestyle and diet improves energy and stress levels almost immediately. And, in the long term, those changes may help protect us from the epidemic of 21st-century diseases now sweeping the Western world. This is what inspired me to write *48 Hours to a Healthier Life*.

I dedicate this book to my Mum and to mums everywhere who spend so much time trying to look after everyone else that they forget to look after themselves.

Introduction

I really mean 48 *waking* hours. Ok, so I cheated – but I had to grab your attention somehow! Forty-eight *waking* hours only equal a long weekend: from Friday lunchtime till Monday lunchtime. One long weekend – that's all I ask you to give yourself as 'me' time. I'm not going to promise you slim, cellulite-free thighs in just three days. But I can promise to get you on the road to a healthier future both physically and emotionally, with cellulite-free thighs thrown in as a long-term benefit!

This book is your home-from-home health spa: it gives you the chance to try out everything you might do at an expensive retreat, but in the comfort of your own home. Apart from saving a heap of money, the main difference is that you can do exactly what you want to do, and when you want to do it. No frantic rushing from one treatment to another. You can eat when you like and sleep when you like and, hopefully, by the end of the Weekend you will want to incorporate many of the techniques and dietary suggestions you have tried into the rest of your life. Everything in the book is affordable and most of the items required are available in larger supermarkets.

This isn't an unrealistic, exclusive plan available only to the few who can fork out for it. It's not about exercising madly for four days, living on carrot juice, and hitting the scales on

Monday one kilo lighter and none the wiser. What it is is *your* time. Whether you're a busy mum, a career girl or a student, *anyone* can find just one weekend in a year to shut the door and look after themselves for once in their lives. How can you give the best to your children and partner, your job or your studies if you're always running on empty?

Treat this book as your own personal plan. Read it from beginning to end, filling in the quizzes along the way. Then decide how much of it you want to try out before and during the Weekend. You might decide to start changing some of your habits straight away, or you might decide to work up to taking the plunge on a specific date. It doesn't matter whether you spend six days, six weeks or six months building up to the Weekend and your bit of 'me time'. It's up to you. Just do it!

Which of these objectives apply to you? Add any more that you can think of.

short-term objectives: I want to . . .

Feel lighter and brighter.
Sleep better.
Reach my optimum weight.
Have more energy.
Balance my moods.
Have clearer skin.
Increase my mental clarity.
Reduce my stress levels.
Improve my digestion.

long-term objectives

There is only one: to be fit and healthy in older age. Whether it is to look and feel younger, avoid menopausal symptoms or just to live a longer, better life. Creaky joints, heart disease and all the other chronic conditions associated with growing older may be in my genes, but I can avoid them or lessen their effects with the right nutrition and lifestyle!

1 The Philosophy: Natural Nutrition

A programme in a very well-known gardening series on British TV recently started with these words: 'Plants need very little to grow healthy – just water, sunlight and nutrients, just like human beings.' Yet, how many of us treat ourselves as well as the plants we cultivate so lovingly? 'Water, sunlight and nutrients' just about sum up what Natural Nutrition is all about – looking after yourself by getting as close to nature as possible.

> 'Natural' means not controlled by man; the wild, primitive state untouched by man or civilization; unspoilt scenery or countryside; the normal biological needs or urges of the body.
>
> 'Nutrition' comes from the Latin 'nutrire', which means to nourish, and from 'nutrix', which means a nurse!

Natural Nutrition has nothing to do with dieting – we know diets do not work in the long term. But it has everything to do with giving your body the very best nutrition you can – four-star petrol and high-grade oil so that the body just runs and runs! So for the Weekend Plan, and hopefully the rest of your life, you're going to give yourself a gold-star service. You're going to nurture your body, mind, spirit and, most importantly, your cells. For without healthy cells you can't have a healthy body or a happy mind. They're the very basis of your well-being and determine how efficiently you function, so we need to understand how they work, and why you need to give them the very best nutrition, fluids and treats!

cells

We have trillions of these – anything from 30 to 100 trillion, no one is absolutely sure! Each of us is just a huge bunch of cells, and every single one of them carries out a valuable job. They protect us from invading bacteria and viruses, cleanse us of toxins and debris using the lymph, and continually regenerate, some at a frightening rate. Eye cells are completely replaced by new ones within 48 hours; but liver cells take six weeks to replicate.

Body cells are very similar in structure to the cells in a gaol! A cell is surrounded by a wall – a fatty membrane that allows in nutrients and substances small enough to filter through its narrow bars. But not everything gets through. And, much like prisoners in a gaol, cells communicate with each other and pass on information about stress, pain, toxicity or even happiness. If they can't communicate with each other *dis-ease* (not disease, but *un-ease*) sets in, and they become dark, cold and rigid, and nothing works quite as it should. At the very least we may experience constipation, bloating, skin problems or headaches. And, at worst, real disease may set in.

> **Sick cells = sick organs and sick organs = disease!**
> **Healthy cells = cleansed organs and cleansed organs = optimum health (and no cellulite)!**

But we're about to change all that this Weekend and make our cells sing and vibrate with energy and happiness!

what we are going to give our cells this weekend for optimum health!

1. Electrolyte Balance
2. Better Nutrition
3. Cleansing
4. More Water
5. The Good Fats
6. Lots of Natural Light
7. Better Breathing
8. Freedom from Stress
9. Relaxation

1. electrolyte balance

Electrolytes are the mineral salts that transport electrical currents in and out of each cell. Think of all those trillions of cells carrying electrical charges constantly, much like a car battery every time the engine is turned over. Except all your cells are turning over 24 hours a day! So if you want to feel like a 'live wire', the electrolyte balance in your body has to be as finely tuned as you can get it.

Very simply put, the four main minerals that will ensure optimum cell health and therefore homeostasis – the perfect balance of fluid and electrolytes throughout the body – are *sodium*, *calcium*, *potassium* and *magnesium*. An upset in equilibrium causes stress and poor functioning at a cellular level. If you've ever read the packet of a rehydration medicine when you've had a bad tummy bug you'll have seen much made of the electrolyte balance.

In everyday rude health, sodium, calcium, potassium and magnesium travel in and out of all the cells, in perfect harmony, day and night. Or they should do! Magnesium and potassium are primarily intracellular nutrients – they should mostly stay *inside* the cell – while calcium and sodium are mostly extra-cellular – they should be *outside* the cells.

Calcium and magnesium work together to regulate the blood, nerves, muscles and tissues in your body. Sodium and potassium help create the electrical charge that makes your muscles and nerves fire on all cylinders. To promote all of this, the four minerals need to move through the cell membranes easily and effortlessly. That movement ensures that the body is always cleansing and finding its own balance.

The trouble is, our 21st-century diet is abundant in calcium and sodium but seriously lacking in magnesium and potassium, so most of the time that perfect flow and balance doesn't exist. The cells become unhappy and don't function or cleanse properly. And every single cell in the body needs to cleanse properly if we are to lose weight, get over illness, and have a healthy, symptom-free body. A 1994 report from the Ministry of Agriculture, Fisheries and Food included statistics that *72 per cent* of women in the UK are seriously deficient in mag-nesium and *as many as 94 per cent* are seriously deficient in potassium.

During the 48-Hour Plan we're going to make sure the cells' electrolyte balance is improved by giving them mag-nesium- and potassium-rich foods but cutting right down on sodium- and calcium-rich foods. Don't worry: you'll get quite enough of both sodium and calcium, in their natural form, from the suggested menus, and it's worth bearing in mind that our hunter-gatherer forefathers managed to get more than 1,000 milligrams of calcium a day – without drinking any milk!

2. better nutrition

Our diet has altered more in the last 50 years than in the last 2,000 years. Since industrialization, our food has changed beyond recognition – and at an accelerated pace over the last two generations. Technology today means that processed foods can be refined, made much tastier by the addition of large quantities of salt, sugar or fat, and stored for months.

And although this high-fat, high-protein diet has made us taller, bigger and generally more 'Amazonian' than ever before, it has not necessarily made us any healthier. In the Western world, we may not suffer from malnutrition and diseases like rickets, but according to the World Health Organization the rates of diabetes, obesity and heart disease are now doubling every decade. Professor Graham MacGregor of St George's Hospital, Tooting, highlights the impact 21st-century living is having on us: 'The commonest cause of death and disability is from heart disease, and the second commonest is from cancer. These diseases are mainly caused by our appalling diet and lifestyle; and if we changed these we would live longer, and also have an enhanced quality of life as we grow older by avoiding unnecessary suffering and enjoying a healthier life.'

Historically, humans started off as nomads and hunter-gatherers – not couch potatoes slumped in front of the TV with a takeaway. Forty thousand years ago we roamed around the land, moving with the seasons, much like some wildlife still does today. We ate the food that was available close by, wherever we were. We were always ready for action with energy on-tap to fight off an attack or kill our next meal. Small meals or snacks were eaten every two to three hours throughout the day. A handful of nuts and seeds gave us our healthy oils, a couple of pieces of fruit or some berries gave us a quick sugar fix, and raw plants and vegetables were as complex a carbohydrate as we ever ate. We caught wild animals such as boar, deer or fish. But we didn't catch them every day. Archaeologists have discovered that we were healthy then, with strong bones and lean, muscular bodies. Yes, we died from simple infections, in childbirth or from accidents. But we didn't die of heart disease or cancer!

For just three days we're going to become more 'gatherers' than 'hunters' with a diet high in raw, fresh food, a few grains and without any animal products. As much as possible, the food we'll be eating will be in season and will have been grown in the country that we live in. After the Weekend, we can revert to being hunter-gatherers, with a lot more protein thrown in. But for 48 hours we are going to concentrate on the foods and techniques that help us cleanse and heal: naturally.

3. cleansing

Detoxing is like 'taking time off work'; it gives the body a chance to cleanse and is a bit like cleaning and oiling a piece of machinery, inside and out, so it will work better and last longer! Resting the digestion allows energy that would usually be used to break down food to be redirected to the cells and tissues, so they can repair themselves by cleansing. Cleansing allows the lymph, blood and organs to clear out old, defective or diseased cells and unneeded chemicals. As the new healthy cells grow, the organs start regenerating and our level of immunity, vitality and disease resistance just soars! Over the Weekend, you're going to try some techniques to boost your body's cleansing capacity.

4. more water

Cells need water – they are 75 per cent water. So water is going to figure as one of the most important requirements of the Weekend Plan. You're probably sick to death of hearing how important water is for your body, but even scientists are now telling us we are dehydrated and need to drink more water.

Dr Susan Shirreffs is an expert on rehydration and a research scientist and lecturer at the Biomedical Sciences Department at Aberdeen University. 'Even small levels of dehydration can create headaches, lethargy or just an overall lack of alertness,' she says. And at a cellular level being dehydrated can be far more serious, claims Dr Shirreffs. 'In the long term it can create problems with the renal system (kidneys) and our mental functioning, as well as our cardiovascular system.'

So start drinking more water from now on!

5. the good fats

Essential fatty acids (EFAs) make up the membranes of every single cell in your body and so influence the state of your health. They control how well your cells cope with what is flowing in and out of them – oxygen, fluid, waste and viruses.

Within each cell are receptor sites where vital hormones, such as insulin, and essential neurotransmitters, such as serotonin, communicate. If the cell membranes are too rigid because of a lack of EFAs, the chemicals can't dock and deliver their messages. The result can be dramatic. With these two examples, you could get blood-sugar blues from an insulin imbalance, and depression because of a shortage of serotonin.

The two essential fatty acids that our bodies need are: linolenic (Omega 3) and linoleic (Omega 6) acids. *All EFAs must come from our food – our bodies can't manufacture them.* But because of our modern eating habits, most of us are seriously deprived of them – especially Omega 3, which is needed in highly concentrated amounts for our brain cells, eyes, adrenal glands and nerves. Without EFAs, we can't produce prostaglandins, the hormone-like group of molecules vital to our well-being. Prostaglandins affect blood pressure, metabolism, nerve impulses and immunity, and control inflammation.

So the Weekend diet will ensure that you're boosting your intake of EFAs. You won't want to live without them once you feel the benefits – it's that instant!

6. lots of natural light

As we've noted, cells pass messages to each other. They also need colour and light to assist communication. If you're keen on holistic treatments, you'll have heard about *chakras* (centres of energy) which, according to yogis and many therapists, sit behind the endocrine glands, where your hormones are produced. Each chakra corresponds to a particular colour and each one needs light. Many therapists also think of cells as mini endocrine systems – so you can see why they believe that wearing bright colours and getting plenty of natural light make the cells – and you – feel so good!

On a more conventional scientific level, there is one chemical message that every single cell in your body is able to receive, the hormone *melatonin* – produced by the brain in response to the amount of sunlight we're exposed to. Melatonin is also a derivative of serotonin, the 'good mood' hormone. During the daylight hours the brain's pineal gland releases very little melatonin, but as darkness falls the levels secreted increase to help the body's internal clock get ready for sleep. In the morning the melatonin production drops off again, and the whole cycle repeats itself. The more bright sunlight you enjoy during the day, the more melatonin will be produced when it gets dark, and the better you'll sleep and feel!

On the other hand, a *shortage* of bright natural light, and therefore a decreased melatonin production, causes many people to suffer from Seasonal Affective Disorder (SAD) and depression during the short winter days. The pineal gland also gets very confused when you travel from one time zone to another, so getting as much natural light as possible when you arrive, no matter what time your body *thinks* it is, will help you adjust to local time, and minimize jet lag.

It's important to know that this amazing chemical – present in all our cells – also assists in maintaining the body's hormonal balance and strengthens immunity, as well as controlling your internal body clock. Therefore, for the sake of your cells, during the three days of the Plan you'll be encouraged to get as much natural daylight as possible.

7. better breathing

Breathing is something we all do, all the time, without thinking – 16 times a minute and using around 13,500 litres (about 3,000 gallons) of air a day! But again, because we are all rushing around, busy and stressed, most of us aren't breathing deeply enough to treat our cells to enough of that essential 'vitamin O', oxygen, without which we have no life or, at the very least, no energy. It's free, everyone can have lots, and this Weekend we're going to learn how to get the best out of this life-saving vitamin for healthier cells and brain and more energy.

It's not just lack of water and missing out on the right fats that can affect our cells and stop them producing optimum health for us. All sorts of outside influences can cause havoc internally and stress our cells – from unhealthy relationships to excessive travel, from a lack of exercise to over-exercising.

As well as affecting every cell in our body, and therefore our overall health, stress can also specifically affect our digestion – big time. In our primitive hunter-gatherer state, when we were under attack from wild beasts we produced adrenaline, a hormone needed for 'fight or flight'. Adrenaline dramatically affects your body in a number of ways, including raising your heart and breathing rates, and increasing your metabolism. At the same time the blood supply to the bladder and intestines is reduced. Nowadays, every time we get stressed – because the kids are playing up, or we have a fit of road rage in the car – valuable blood is being shunted away from our organs, such as the brain or intestines, and sent to our muscles so we are made ready to run away or stand our ground and fight! Because we're not actively fighting or fleeing packs of wolves any more, all that stress from modern living stays in our body; this affects our gut, causing food intolerances, digestive problems and a toxic build-up. All of which will depress our immune system and make us ill if left unchecked.

Stress = a run-down immune system = dis-ease.

Apart from diet, one of the best ways to help our bodies and cells get over stress is exercise. We were built to move around constantly: to plough, plant and harvest, or hunt our food. This weekend we will be getting off our bottoms and moving around a lot more than normal – preferably outside where the light can benefit us.

9. relaxation

Relaxation is also an essential part of tackling stress. I often think, especially in the UK where we have the longest working hours in Europe, that we're just like hamsters on a wheel going round and round and round without stopping for breath. Our cells need rest to recuperate, and getting rid of tension in the body by relaxing for as little as 10–20 minutes a day can be almost as good as a night's sleep for cell regeneration.

> **We are human 'beings', not 'doings', so for the 48-Hour Plan we are going to learn how to 'be' again to lead a healthier life!**

So if we feel like sleeping for 14 hours a night over the Weekend, we can do that too! Before electricity we would have slept for 12–14 hours a night in the winter; there was little else to do. So, as we're going back to nature, for just three days anything goes – as long as it's natural.

But, first, let's spend some time looking at how you can build up gradually and gently to the Weekend.

2. Preparing for Your Weekend

START NOW! It doesn't matter whether you decide to do your 48-Hour Plan in six days', six weeks' or even six months' time. To avoid the potholes of cravings, mood swings and withdrawal symptoms, you might like to start walking along the road to a healthier life right now, and build up slowly and gently to the big Weekend.

In this chapter, we're going to consider:

Who you want to spend the 48-Hour Detox Weekend with, if anybody.

What you're going to be encouraged to do without during that weekend and what you might like to try cutting out now.

Why it's important for you to do this plan.

Where you're going to spend your three days.

When might be the best time to start detoxing for minimum withdrawal symptoms and maximum impact.

who?

Who should you spend this Weekend with? There's no question that the effects of a cleansing weekend, on both body and mind, are much stronger if the time is spent in quiet solitude, with *just you* for company. Having done it by myself, I can only beg you to try – because turning the world off and shutting down the outside chatter is a bit like taking your brain out and giving it a good rinse! The three-day break feels as if you have had a week's holiday, with the added bonus of having been healthy *and* utterly self-indulgent. But you need to know what sort of person you are and if you can cope on your own. If you've never spent a night away from your partner or have never been on holiday on your own, then doing it solo isn't for you.

If you have a dog, or can borrow one, you may well decide that this is the best compromise of all. A dog won't tempt you to open a bottle of wine, and you'll get lots of fresh air and exercise. And if you're not used to spending much time alone, pets – even borrowed ones – are fantastic company and make you feel secure at night – and they don't talk!

If you really want human contact there are several options. Many women I meet are so enthusiastic about the Plan that they decide to spend a cheap weekend away with a girl friend, leaving their husbands to have some 'quality time' with the kids at home! You could rent a cottage, borrow a friend's flat, or do a house swap with each other – sending dads and kids to one home, while the two of you get down to the Plan in the other home, without any distractions. Any arrangement you like, as long as it's self-catering. Think of the fun dad could have with the kids. They could go off to do things together that they've never had the chance to do before, such as camping, fishing, visiting a theme park, playing football and golf, and so on. (Having read that list, I think if I was a daughter I would want to stay at home with mum!)

If you decide to spend the Weekend with a friend, the *who* is very important: it needs to be someone as dedicated to the experience as you, and not the sort of person who is going to lead you astray on the first evening with temptations of 'just one tiny little drinkie'. She (or he) also needs to be someone who is happy to try just sitting and being 'still and silent' for 10 minutes at a time without being embarrassed and bursting into giggles. Someone you can be completely honest with, someone with whom you can discuss your bowel movements, or how lousy you feel. Someone who is used to seeing you without any make-up and in scruffy clothes or a dressing gown. The sort of friend or companion you have shared your innermost thoughts and secrets with!

That person could well be your husband or partner, and I can't think of a better way to re-evaluate your relationship and renew your sex life. If you spend a long weekend together learning massage techniques, turning the TV off, and without the kids, you can't fail to find out how you're both feeling about your life together. But it's a brave move and not for the faint-hearted!

So sit and have a think now about who you might like to spend this Weekend with and why they are suitable. But don't make any final decisions till you have finished reading the book, and then come back to this page and fill in the form.

WHO	BENEFITS	DRAWBACKS
Just Me	No one else to think about.	Can't sleep in the house alone.
Pets		
Best girl friend		
Partner		
Daughter		
Sister		
Mother		
A.N. Other (gay male friend, yoga-loving male friend, etc.)		

what?

Have a look at the CRAVINGS LIST below and tick the things that ring a bell. It's probably the most telling list in the whole book. I don't usually need to do intolerance testing when I see clients, because simply asking them what they crave and what they can't imagine living without is the single biggest clue to any intolerance they may be suffering from. Very few people crave seeds, nuts, water, fruit or vegetables! Come to think of it, when did you last see a saucy advert for pumpkin seeds? Everyone's list inevitably includes bread and pasta, or chocolate, or coffee, or alcohol, or all four. Go ahead, you try it now.

- Cigarettes
- Alcohol
- Sugar
- Tea
- Coffee
- Dairy: Milk and Cheese
- Bread
- Cakes, Pastries, Biscuits
- Chocolate
- Sweets
- Sweet Fizzy Drinks, whether low calorie or not
- Salty Snacks like Crisps, whether low fat or not
- Fried Food
- Meat
- Takeaways
- Processed Food

How did you do?

You might like to start thinking about cutting right back very soon on one of the items you've ticked. If you reduce your intake of things you can't imagine living without *gradually*, and only one at a time, your body won't go into shock, with symptoms like a detoxing headache, bloating or skin eruptions. Pick a day when you feel particularly rested, strong and full of good intentions, and decide either to cut back on your intake slowly and gradually or, if you're feeling really brave, give something up altogether. And do that with every 'tick', one a week, till you're eating or drinking the very minimum quantities of all of them. Remember that you don't need to give up your 'ticks' *completely*, just cut down to such a degree that doing without them for three days is not going to cause you a massive problem.

If you want to give something up gradually, look at this

example: you might at the moment be in the habit of drinking 6–8 cups of tea a day, with milk and sugar or sweetener. Start in **week 1** by halving the number of cups of tea you usually drink. In **week 2** halve it again. In **week 3** halve the amount of sugar; in **week 4** drop the sugar completely. By **week 5** start trying to do without the milk, and then eventually you'll be down to 1–2 cups of black tea a day. Without the milk and sugar, you probably won't enjoy the tea half as much, so it'll be much easier to cut down on the number of cuppas. If you *can't* drink it black, don't worry – it's more important to try and get past the sugar craving than give up dairy products at this point. You do *not* want sugar or artificial sweeteners in your diet at any time in the future, for the sake of your health and your weight, so this would be a really good place to start.

targets for cutting down or giving up an addiction
(be it 3 alcoholic drinks a night, or 20 ciggies a day, or a bar of chocolate every tea time.)

WEEK 1	Halve the amount.
WEEK 2	Halve the intake again.
WEEK 3	One small portion a day.
WEEK 4	Try and have it once a week only.

Work out your own plan, with your own diary, so it's really manageable for you and you alone. Or agree to do it with a friend for encouragement and support. (If you think you'll have trouble giving something up, try to start the process on a Friday – or Friday evening – so you have the weekend to deal with any symptoms or a bad mood!)

the one thing I want you to have **more** of: water!

One thing I really need you to change from now on, even if you do nothing else, is to start drinking more water, building up to 2 litres (3½ pints) of water – just eight large glasses – a day.

At this juncture, I don't care if it's bottled fizzy or bottled still, or tap water. I just need you to drink common-or-garden plain, unflavoured water in bigger quantities than you're used to, from now on. It'll help you get over any cravings, keep your blood-sugar levels even, stop mood swings and fill you up. And you'll look and feel much, much better – I promise!

why?

Why are you doing this Weekend? Yes, part of the plan is to encourage you to follow a healthier diet, to detox and cleanse, and maybe even lose a little weight. But, just as importantly, the Weekend will also calm your whole nervous system and de-stress your mind. To reiterate: getting you off that hamster wheel and giving your brain and body a good clear-out. All of which will benefit the health of your mind, body and spirit for the long term (and for ever if you continue with just a few of the book's suggestions).

You'll also be stimulating all five of your senses this weekend: *hearing*, *seeing*, *tasting*, *touching* and *smelling*. Recent research entitled 'The Secrets of the Senses' (published by I C I and Oxford University) reports that most of us are suffering from sensory deprivation – and that this is affecting our health. For the last 100 years scientists have treated each sense separately. But, after a decade of multi-sensory research, Experimental Psychologist and Cognitive Neuro Scientist Dr Charles Spence, the author of the report, confirms for the first time that the five senses are integrated and should work together, not separately.

According to Dr Spence, 21st-century living under-uses our *emotional* senses but we're suffering from a visual and auditory overload! 'We're spending 90 per cent of our time indoors, watching TV or sitting in front of a computer,' warns Dr Spence. 'We're neglecting our two most important *emotional* senses – touch and smell – and this imbalance is negatively affecting our health and well-being.'

In fact, according to the research, personal pampering is a virtue and not a vice, and you may actually improve your productivity and efficiency if you spend a little time on nurturing those unfulfilled senses – touch and smell. So you can now wallow, guilt-free, in a scented bath, give yourself a massage, and know this is actually benefiting your health. But, in order to stimulate those neglected senses, the TV has to go!

Some of you will think it's not possible to live without a television or a mobile phone. (I was one of those people!) *But it is only for three days and it will change your life for ever*. (And to make it easier you can always find somewhere cheap to stay for the 48-Hour Plan that has no mobile signal and a poor TV reception!)

In preparation for the Weekend, look at this list of things that we all do or use that could be causing us stress and sapping our energy – things that we need to cut down on and eventually eliminate as much as possible during the three days, if we're to get back to a natural state of bliss.

stressers and energy sappers

Mobile phone and texting
Ordinary phone
Watching TV
Listening to the radio or
   music – unless it's
   soothing!

Driving the car
Using the computer
Using a fax machine
Wearing a watch
Alarm clock

During the weeks leading up to the Weekend, start spending just one day a week, or just half a day a week, or one evening a week, without one or all of those *stressers*. Treat it as an experiment. Go on, try it!

We *can* live without these things because we used to, quite happily. Mobiles, e-mail, fax machines, computers, personal organizers are all wonderful hi-tech things that are supposed to make our lives easier. While it's certainly easier for me now to write this book than it would have been 30 years ago, there's no doubt that we work much longer hours and are more stressed than ever before. We're now accessible to anyone and everyone 24/7, and that in itself can be very stressful.

ways to start reducing stress levels before the weekend

- 10 minutes a day fast walking outside in the light, no matter what the weather!
- 10 minutes a day spent doing absolutely nothing, thinking of nothing, in silence. (Do it in the bathroom if that is your only means of escape.)
- 10 minutes a day spent cooking, or gardening, or anything manual without any 'noise' on.

- 5 minutes a day spent stretching. (See exercises in chapter 10.)
- 5 minutes a day spent on skin-brushing. (See chapter 6.)

where?

The *who* section may well dictate *where* you might be going, if anywhere, to do your 48-Hour Plan. You may be sharing your home with a friend, or renting a cottage together in the country, or borrowing a friend's flat. It doesn't really matter where it is as long as it's self-catering, and you can control the environment and the fuel that goes into your body. Hotels and B&Bs are out of the question – there are too many distractions and temptations!

But if you're spending the weekend with a friend or partner, it might be an idea to find out what you both need in the way of outside influences. What will really help you both relax? Is there a big park near either of your homes, or a river, or the sea? Can you get peace and quiet outside as well as inside?

Personally, I need to be near water as often as possible. I am a Scorpio, so I crave being by water, especially the sea. So for me the ultimate detox would be spent on the coast without leaving the country. Others need to be surrounded by trees; some people like mountains and lakes, and some just don't want to leave home. In fact, the first time I did the 48-Hour Plan, I found it much easier to do in my own home because everything was at hand and it felt comfortable. The next time, I went to Cornwall, where there was absolutely no signal on my mobile and a terrible reception on both TV and radio – so that worked too!

Try this simple exercise now to see which is the location to get the best benefits from your Weekend away. Just sit quietly without the TV or radio on, somewhere private such as the bathroom, and try and empty your mind for five minutes. Now take a piece of paper and a pen, and draw a circle with seven branches coming out of it. Put the word WEEKEND in the circle and, without giving yourself a chance to think, tap your subconscious by writing the first seven words or phrases that pop into your mind, very quickly, one word or phrase on each of the branches. It's just like a word-association game, but is called 'mind-mapping' and is something I have found invaluable for studying, making life decisions and even writing this book. It'll help you find out what your inner self really needs (unless you know already!).

Here's how mine looked:

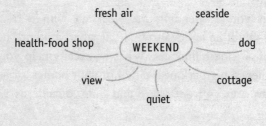

What'll be on yours?

when?

Because you may need plenty of time to eliminate foods that doing without could cause you a problem over the three days, your Weekend may need to be planned well in advance in your diary. Also, the seasons and even the moon cycles, believe it or not, can play a major part in whether it's going to be really tough or relatively easy to stick to the Plan. The more foods you want to exclude, the longer you need as a build-up and the harder it will be to exclude them all. So take your time and do take the seasons, the moon, and whatever else might help you into account! I don't want you to feel terrible for the entire three days! It's supposed to be a positive experience.

On the other hand, if you're already matching many of my recommendations on diet and fluids intake, you may well be able to just plunge right in and follow the Plan almost immediately. Remember: you can start in six days, six weeks or even six months. The choice is yours – decide on when according to your own circumstances and habits.

seasons

Spring is truly a season for new beginnings. Everything is renewed, plants, trees, animals – all are thriving. The earth's energy really surges at this time of year and it's one of the best times to start a detox and introduce a new eating plan for life. The body is happier with cleansing foods like smoothies, raw vegetables and salads, fruit, seeds and nuts. The closer it gets to *summer*, the less we need in the way of 'stodgy' foods, and the easier it will be to improve your eating habits. Your sleep patterns change as well, and you should find yourself waking up earlier – naturally.

Summer is when we should reach up to the sun for our nourishment, just like the garden does. Being outside sustains us, and our food should be as colourful as our flowers! This is the easiest time of the year to lose weight and get up early, as we're feeling more active.

Autumn is another time when the body is really receptive to a change in eating patterns. It is, along with *spring*, the most beneficial time to cleanse as the body prepares itself for winter. Many people find they get fewer colds or bouts of flu and don't suffer from SAD (Seasonal Affective Disorder) during the winter months if they have prepared themselves for the shorter days by eating nutritious, cleansing foods. This is a time for much warmer foods – steamed vegetables, soups and hot drinks. We'll be heading indoors, and we'll want to sleep more – and so we should!

Winter: We need more fuel for our body's furnace and more sleep to recharge our batteries (and our thoughts turn to 'hibernating' in our caves!). This is the time of the year to catch as many catnaps as we can – if only work or the kids would allow us to!

NEW YEAR, NEW START

Of course the time that most of us want to start a detox plan and swap old habits for new is the worst possible month – January. It's one of the hardest times of the year for the body to cleanse because it has its work cut out just keeping you healthy fighting all the viruses around. On the other hand, this is the best time of the year to give up things like alcohol and cigarettes, because everyone else is trying to. It's also a very good time for locking yourself away and being 'quiet' as the pressure of socializing eases right off after the Christmas festivities.

Whichever season you decide on to start your 48-Hour Plan, there will be plenty of meal suggestions appropriate for that time of the year. You'll find recipes in chapter 17.

moon cycles

The moon affects the tides, our monthly cycles and even the birth rate. Did you know that many midwives and hospitals are on standby for a rise in birth rates during a full moon? The reason is simple. Inside every cell in our bodies there is a pull and a push going on in synch with the moon's rhythms, just like the ebb and flow of the tide. There is even a tide in that glass of water sitting in front of you. (Drink up!)

During the *full moon* the pull of the moon on those tides is stronger than at any other time – hence a high tide, violent storms and people going a bit loony. Have you ever noticed how bloated you feel around a full moon? Check it out next time, it's your cells heading for a high tide!

It's hardly surprising then that the moon is going to have a profound effect on the *cleansing* ability of our bodies. On a *new* moon the pull on the cells is much weaker and less dramatic, much like a low tide, so side effects and withdrawal symptoms will be kept to a minimum. (And ovulating is associated with a *new* moon, so you might want to tuck that one away if you are trying for a baby!) So, as wacky as it sounds, if it's proving really difficult for you to give up finally coffee, cigarettes or alcohol, make sure you pick a new moon day to do it. Mentally as well as physically a new moon is associated with new beginnings.

What's the best time to do the Weekend? As the moon travels from full to new – a waning moon – it's much easier, and more beneficial, for the body to detoxify and cleanse during those two weeks. The closer to the date of the new moon the more effective your attempt will be. But any time during the fortnight *following* a full moon will be suitable, so check your diary – most of them have the moon cycles listed.

stocking up

You may well have an idea of when, where and with whom you'll want to do the 48-Hour Plan. You might even be starting to cut down on some of your cravings, internal and external. Soon you'll be feeling strong enough to incorporate all the Plan for three days.

But, first, here's a checklist of the non-food items you'll need for your Weekend. You may have many of them already, and if you stock up gradually by adding the smaller items to your weekly shop bit by bit, the expenditure won't hurt as much. Most major supermarkets now have a 'health section' where you will find many of the basics you'll need. Others will be stocked in high-street health shops. For the bigger and more expensive items, you may want to ask friends and family to buy you one of them as a birthday or Christmas present.

non-food basics

Water Filter

Blender (Any inexpensive one, it doesn't need to be state of the art.)

Juicer (There are cheap ones on sale, but a juicer isn't essential unless you're doing a spring or summer detox.)

Hand-Held Shower Attachment

Cozy Dressing Gown

Fluffy Towels

Yoga Mat or Floor Mat

3 small packets (3 × 200 gr/½ lb) of Epsom Salts

Body Brush

Face Flannel

Loofah

Natural Sponge

Your choice of Carrier and Essential Oils to use for self-massage (see chapter 6) and in baths (see chapter 8)

Oil Burner

Candles

Joss Sticks

Classical or New-Age Music on CD or cassette (and portable CD or cassette player if going away)

You may also want to start stocking up on some of the more unusual non-perishable foods on the list. Again, if you start popping them into your trolley during your weekly shop, you won't notice the extra expense.

non-perishables to start stocking up on (organic wherever possible)

MUST-HAVES (unless you have an allergy)

Almonds, Brazil Nuts, Walnuts, Cashews, Chestnuts – any nuts, apart from peanuts, and as long as they're unsalted.

Golden Linseeds (Flaxseeds)

Linseed Oil (Keep in fridge)

Sesame, Pumpkin and Sunflower Seeds and Pine Nuts (Keep in fridge)

Lecithin Granules

Short-Grain Brown Rice or Basmati Brown Rice

Green Tea or other Herbal Teas

Aloe Vera Juice – an anti-inflammatory cleanser I would strongly recommend. Keep it in the fridge.

OPTIONALS

Tick items off as you buy them, concentrating on the ones you know you like (as opposed to buying things that you think you *should* like!). Once you've read the book through you'll have a better idea of which techniques and recipes (see chapter 17) you're likely to want to try, and then start stocking up on all those optional bits and pieces you'll need.

Bottled Water

Light Tahini Paste (the lightest, runniest one you can find)

Clear Honey

Tinned Chickpeas and other Pulses

Dried Lentils

Tinned Tomatoes

Sundried Tomatoes

Vegetable Stock Cubes

Olives

Oatmeal

Your choice of Grain Alternatives (see chapter 5)

Sea Salt

Tamari (a salt substitute made from soya beans)

Nori Flakes (a salt substitute from the sea) or other Sea Vegetable
    Flavouring

Brown Rice Vinegar – this is more natural and less fermented
    than ordinary vinegars but Apple Cider Vinegar will do.

Sesame Oil (for the teeth)

Mustard/Mustard Powder

Olive Oil

Soya or Rice Milk

Coconut Milk

Dried Apricots and Figs

Dried Spices: Chilli, Cayenne, Cinnamon, Turmeric, Cumin Seeds
    or Garam Masala

Spirulina or Wheat Grass – supplements in powder form that
    contain high levels of nutrients and are useful in a detox.

fresh food shopping

When you've checked the meal suggestions, you'll have a good
idea of what fresh produce you'll need for the Weekend. All I
can say is, Have plenty of fruit and vegetables! (There's a lot
more information on the merits of fruit and veg in chapter 5.)
But I leave the choice largely to you. Certainly, lemons, fresh
garlic, ginger and herbs are pretty essential. For some of the

more exotic ingredients, such as galangal (a lovely sweet ginger used in Thai cooking) you might want to try out your local Indian or Thai shops.

preparation checklist – have I . . . ?

- Decided who is joining me for the weekend.
- Cut down on my addictions.
- Started drinking more water.
- Tried a day without the 'stressers'.
- Decided where to go.
- Checked seasons against my food preferences.
- Checked moon cycles.
- Checked for a weekend with no social engagements.
- Checked the long-range weather forecast.
- Started buying items on the shopping lists.
- Made sure I am ready for this.

Are you ready for the first stage? Drinking more water – much more water! The next chapter will explain why this is so important, which type is the best, and how much is the right amount.

3. H for H$_2$O – Water!

Three-quarters of the earth's surface is water, and the same goes for our bodies. Between 65 and 75 per cent of a living human being is made up of water – slopping around in our blood, tissues, organs and bones. All of it is absolutely vital for the body to carry out its many functions.

so what does water do in the body?

- Water carries oxygen to every single cell in the body. It also transports sodium, calcium, magnesium, potassium and other salts in and out through the cell membranes to achieve electrolyte balance, without which nothing functions as well as it should.
- When there's enough water in the body, the blood and lymphatic fluid can flow more easily. The blood carries enzymes and nutrients to the organs, and the lymph fluid connects with the bloodstream to take waste away to the elimination routes (skin, nose, bowel, kidneys and lungs).
- Water helps dilute acids in the body, making the blood more alkaline and the internal system healthier. It also moisturizes the skin, making it look younger, and is essential for brain health. We sometimes forget that the brain is an organ too – an organ

that is almost entirely made up of water and fat. A watery fluid cushions every joint and bone in the body and every single vertebra is also surrounded by it, so if you want a healthy, pain-free back, *get drinking*!

- Without water we would have no saliva, mucous membranes or digestive juices. Water also helps regulate our body's temperature and maintains blood-glucose levels by releasing sugar from the cells as needed. (Try drinking a couple of glasses of water next time you're hungry and can't get to any food.)

- Finally, many therapists, including me, believe *dis-ease* starts in the colon (the lower part of the large intestine) and the colon is where the body uses a huge percentage of its water intake to bulk up the waste and help move it along and out of the body. The more water you drink, the more frequently you will move your bowels, and the less waste and toxicity will be left behind to fester in the body.

And (briefly) even more benefits of drinking water

Helps kidneys excrete acids.
Relieves stress.
Reduces cholesterol levels.
Helps blood pressure.
Prevents headaches.

Prevents hangovers (!)
Prevents fatigue.
Helps prevent allergic reactions.

but won't other fluids do?

In a word: NO! Something I like to ask people who don't drink water is, 'If you have a dog or cat, what's the first thing you check in the morning or when you get home in the evening?'

The water bowl. 'And if you have a garden or just a few plants around your flat, what do you give them?' *Water.*

Some dogs *do* enjoy a bowl of beer – *occasionally*. Some gardeners swear by putting tea leaves on their plants – *occasionally*. And some cats love a saucer of cream – *very occasionally*. But, as their main fluid, they all need *water* 90 per cent of the time. And so do we.

We can still drink coffee, tea, wine, beer, etc., in moderation (BUT NOT DURING THE WEEKEND PLAN!). But for a healthy body and mind we need to increase our intake of water to make up for drinking liquids that aren't actually giving us anything we need, except a great deal of psychological comfort! Well, *OK*, there *are* rich antioxidants in some wines and teas, but these are still diuretics, which overwork our kidneys. Colas and soft drinks should be considered VERY, VERY RARELY, if at all. (But more on that later.) Rehydration expert Dr Susan Shirreffs explains, 'Tea, coffee, cola or anything that contains caffeine may act as a diuretic and stimulate urination of fluid. Alcohol has an even stronger diuretic effect than caffeine.' In other words, every time you drink a cup of coffee or tea or a glass of alcohol, you're encouraging your kidneys to take *out of your body* more fluid than you have just put in.

> **Too many diuretics in a day cause stress to the body, and stress causes dehydration.**

Have a look at this list and tick any symptoms that apply to you.

dehydration symptoms checklist

- Dark Yellow Urine
- Constipation
- Tired All the Time
- Bad Skin
- Hungry All the Time
- Mood Swings

- Hormonal Problems
- High Cholesterol
- Backache
- Joint Problems
- Headaches

well, how much water should I drink?

Believe it or not, we lose 2 litres (about 3½ pints) of water from our bodies every day without actually *doing* anything. The water is lost through perspiration, breathing, coughing, sneezing, menstruating, pooing and weeing – just being. So we need to replace that amount of lost water as a bare minimum – even more if you're exercising or leading a very stressful life.

As a matter of course I would recommend at least 1½ to 3 litres (around 2½ to 5 pints) of fluid a day (including fruit juice and other beverages). Certainly, during the Plan, drinking 2 litres of pure, unadulterated water a day is essential if you're to detox safely and happily. That's only eight tumblers of water a day.

You'll know when you're drinking enough by having a quick look at your urine. Apart from first thing in the morning (when your body will be very dehydrated) you need to aim for straw-coloured urine – a very pale yellow.

> **WARNING: Don't drink more than 2 pints (1.1 litres) in one hour. Too much water can upset the electrolyte balance, overwork the kidneys and/or cause the brain to swell.**

but what if I have a weak bladder?

When you first start drinking more water, make sure you pick days when you'll be at home, or somewhere with easy access to a loo. Check that it'll be a couple of weeks before you need to make too many long journeys. But don't worry: your bladder will adapt to the increase in liquid and soon you won't need to keep rushing to the loo to empty it.

It may take a week or two, but as your body becomes more and more used to being 'hydrated' it will want more and more water and you may find, for the first time in your life, that you develop a thirst for it. It happened to me – and I was one of those people who found drinking water 'boring', and who often had to get up in the night to go to the loo. Very soon my body changed. I was surprised to find that I soon 'craved' my glasses of water, and the only thing that got me up at night was if I had been drinking wine or too much coffee during the day!

when should I drink water?

1. Try and stagger your glasses of water throughout the day. It's amazing how much you can get through if you leave a 2-litre bottle out and fill a tumbler every hour on the hour. You don't have to drink the whole glass at once – just take a couple of sips whenever you think of it.

2. If you're worried about getting up in the night, drink your last glass of water before 9 p.m. You'll still have got through 8–10 glasses, and even more if you kick off the day with a glass as soon as you wake up!

3. When it comes to meal times, try *not* to drink water *with* your food as it can interfere with the digestion. Leaving 30 minutes to an hour either side of the meal will help your gut break down the food.

what type of water should I drink?

1. *Still* water rather than fizzy – it's much easier to drink more of it. The bubbles in carbonated water fill you up too quickly, so your natural thirst disappears. Bubbles also make you gassy, bloat the cells and encourage cellulite, so that should convince you!

2. If you have to add a flavouring, don't buy juice in a bottle or carton – get more nutrients and save your money by squeezing a little fresh fruit juice, such as orange or lemon, into a glass of water. *If you must!* This is also a good tip for getting children to drink more water and weaning them off additive- and sugar-packed soft drinks.

3. Water at room temperature is much easier to drink more of as it's close to the body's natural temperature and doesn't shock the stomach like an ice-cold drink would (one of the main reasons people get stomach upsets on holiday in very hot climates).

tap or bottle?

The experts can't agree on this one, so I'm going to leave the decision to you. Within reason, I don't really care as long as you get that water down you! I would rather you were rehydrating your body than worrying about buying the most expensive gadget that takes every single chemical out of the water. But here are some guidelines to help you make your decision.

Tap Water: Usually tastes too disgusting and is often laden with chemicals and minerals – some of them good for you and some of them bad.

Soft Water: Has had most of its minerals removed and is usually high in sodium. So if you live in a soft-water area stay away from the tap!

Hard Water: Usually has more minerals, particularly calcium and magnesium, so at a push this may be ok, provided it tastes half-decent!

! TOP TIP FOR TASTY TAP WATER

If tap water is the only water that suits your budget but it tastes foul, try this. Boil a full kettle of tap water. Leave the water to cool in a big, wide-mouthed non-plastic jug so the air can circulate. When it's cool, pour it into another container from a height of at least 6 inches. And then pour it back into the first jug. Repeat this a couple of times, finishing with the water in that jug. It sounds mad, but it does actually oxygenate the water (something anyone who keeps fish will know about!) and makes it taste better. And it's free!

Natural Mineral Water: By law it has to come from a natural source at which it's bottled, and must have a constant mineral composition. It's not processed so it is, by very definition, natural. BUT check the labels very carefully and make sure it's *low in calcium and sodium*. Remember the electrolyte balance explained in chapter 1.

Spring Water: Can be 'natural' or 'processed' in the UK, but in mainland Europe should only be 'natural'. Again, read the label carefully.

Water from a Jug Filter: The cheapest and easiest home-filter option. Filters are much more affordable than they used to be, but they only filter a limited amount of water at a time, and the filter needs changing regularly. However, it's cheaper and more environmentally friendly than carrying all those plastic bottles home from the shops.

Water from an 'Under-the-Sink' Filter: More expensive than a jug filter, but also uses activated carbon. It's a very effective filter as it takes out herbicides, pesticides, chlorine, 75 per cent of any fluoride in the water, plus lead, copper, cadmium and mercury.

Reverse-Osmosis Process: Even more expensive, but excludes almost 100 per cent of the impurities found in water, including fluoride. However, it also removes virtually all the naturally occurring minerals, some of which may do us some good. There is no need to worry about the lack of minerals, though, if fruit and vegetables are a mainstay of your diet, as you'll get all the minerals you need from those.

Distilled Water: Expensive and the distillation unit takes up space. The jury is out on this one. Some experts say this is the very purest water on the planet because it contains none of the inorganic minerals found in both tap and mineral water and none of the poisons and pollutants found in tap water. Others say it's too pure and it could 'leach' precious minerals out of our bodies just as pure rainwater leaches minerals from the rocks. (Again, your new eating habits will make sure there are plenty of minerals being put back into your body.)

So there you are – your decision. As long as you get it down you I don't think you need to lose sleep over what type of water you're drinking. Choose the method and type that is most convenient to you and your purse! (What do I drink? A mixture of distilled water and shop-bought mineral water that is low in sodium and calcium, and sometimes even tap water if I'm in an area where it tastes nice!)

! **TOP TIPS** FOR DRINKING WATER

Make sure it's still, not fizzy.

Make sure it's at room temperature.

DON'T drink it WITH your meals but drink water 30 minutes before a meal . . . and 1–2 hours after a meal.

DON'T DRINK MORE THAN 2 PINTS (1.1 LITRES) IN AN HOUR.

Don't drink after 9–10 p.m. at night.

Use a bottle to monitor how much water you're drinking. You might not be regularly buying bottled water, but use a clean 2-litre bottle and fill it up at the beginning of the day. Keep it on your desk or kitchen counter, and make sure it's empty by the end of the day!

4 E for **Eliminating** the Challenging Foods

Everything that we eat or drink is foreign to our internal system, until it has been chemically altered and labelled. Put very simply, the mouth and stomach mechanically and chemically break down food into components small enough to be absorbed from the small intestine into the blood. From there those components are taken to the body's chemical factory, the liver, where they are broken down even further and boxed up as 'friend' or 'foe'. Friends are sent off round the body as nutrients, and foes are expelled!

Just imagine that each food poses a different challenge to the body, and the more severe the challenge the more dehydrated and stressed the cells become in processing that food. If the body is constantly challenged over a long period it may become very 'dry' and then the stomach won't be able to digest properly everyday foods such as cheese sandwiches or chocolate, and the liver won't be able to do its job efficiently. 'Challenging' foods take an enormous amount of the digestive system's energy to be broken down and used or thrown out. The more complex the meal the more energy is needed to deal with it, and the more lethargic we feel as our blood is shunted away from places like the brain to go to work in the digestive process.

If the digestion is over-taxed, the gastro-intestinal tract

(your gut) becomes clogged with stagnating food, and the thousands of little finger-like projections in your small intestines (villi) will no longer absorb the food correctly, and *dis-ease* will set in.

Dis-ease, in this context, is acidity in the cells. If the cells are too acidic, they can't get rid of toxins or excess acids easily and won't absorb essential minerals and nutrients. I won't go into minute detail about specific pH levels, but the body produces both acidic and alkaline fluids. The stomach juices should be acidic while bile and pancreatic juice should be alkaline. Together these last two neutralize the stomach's contents as they come through the small intestine. But because of our diet, most of us are acidic in places where we should be alkaline, and alkaline where we should be acidic! Overall, a healthy body should be about 70 per cent alkaline and only 30 per cent acidic. All too often, it's the reverse. And this excess acidity increases the likelihood of our developing illnesses and accelerates ageing. So it's vital to try to redress the balance.

All this is why, for just three days, the exclusion list of no-go foods is pretty strict. Don't worry, there will be plenty of tasty and less challenging alternatives, which will give the body as little to do as possible. So it can concentrate on resting and repairing important organs such as the bowel and liver, and allow its internal environment to become a perfect acidic-alkaline mix – a sort of spring clean of your intestines.

say no to these acidic and challenging foods

The 3 'S's: Sugar, Salt and Stimulants
Dairy Products: Cheese, Milk & Cream
Wheat

Animal Products, including Meat, Fish and Eggs
Potatoes (and Aubergines, Tomatoes, Courgettes and Peppers if
    you suffer from arthritis)

I bet you're looking at this list in blind panic, thinking, What is there left to eat? Don't panic: in the next chapter we'll look at all the alternatives. And do remember: *it is only for three days*! Once you've read the reasons for excluding them, you might even agree (and do it for longer)!

the 3 's's: sugar

Contrary to what we're led to believe by the manufacturers of soda pop, sweets, chocolates and cakes, sugar has absolutely *no* nutritional value whatsoever. Yes, it's lovely and it's moreish. But the fix that can only be satisfied by a mid-afternoon chocolate bar is simply a drop in our blood-sugar levels.

Blood sugar is glucose – our main source of energy without which we couldn't be active. But *refined* sugar, in the form of a biscuit or a sugary drink, makes the blood-sugar levels peak too quickly and, unless you're running a marathon, the glucose produced has nowhere to go. It gets transported to the cells, is dumped there and the body starts laying down fat.

Every time sugar is eaten, the pancreas releases the hormone insulin to cope with the sudden rise in blood-sugar levels. Just half an hour after eating something sugary, we'll want more to repeat that blood-sugar high. And so the roller-coaster ride of extreme blood-sugar highs followed by blood-sugar lows begins. This can lead to headaches, irritability, mood swings, low energy, feeling cold and, eventually, if you're unlucky, insulin resistance. The pancreas is being asked to produce insulin so often it just runs out. And the result could be obesity, diabetes and, in the end, heart disease.

And if that doesn't convince you, this certainly will! Sugar weakens our immune system – big time! In one study, youngsters were given a soft drink that contained 66 grams of sugar. Within *just 45 minutes* their immune cells' ability to engulf bacteria had dropped by *half*.

artificial sweeteners

Artificial sweeteners are the most common and most consumed food additives today. They are cheaper than sugar and some are up to 300 times sweeter. They are also hidden in a great many things other than diet drinks and low-cal foods: crisps and other savoury snacks, ready-made meals and even so-called 'healthy' orange juice. Children are consuming huge amounts of them and no one yet knows the long-term effects on the body. 'We use artificial sweeteners regularly for our patients' weight-loss programmes,' explains Dr Stephen Waring, a specialist in Cardiovascular Risk at the University of Edinburgh. But he adds, 'They haven't been properly researched in a clinical setting and this gives me cause for great concern.'

Obesity has tripled in the last 15 years, yet we're actually eating fewer calories and less fat, and consuming more *diet* colas and drinks than ever before. So they're not working, are they? Most health professionals think there is a link and that low-cal drinks may actually encourage weight *gain* because the taste buds are being conned. They taste 'sugar', the pancreas produces insulin, and off we go again on that roller coaster of wanting more and more sugar which, if it isn't burned off, results in more fat being stashed away.

And most fizzy soft drinks, whether diet or 'full-fat', are loaded with *phosphorus*. Although this mineral is essential for healthy bones, the amount contained in a bottle of pop is so high that it literally drags calcium out of the bones (as the minerals compete for absorption). Add a poor diet to the equation, and you won't be surprised to hear that osteoporosis bone-scan clinics are seeing a huge rise in brittle bones amongst twenty-somethings – because of the amounts of soda pop they're drinking. So if you want brittle bones, just carry on drinking a litre of low-cal fizzy a day!

Remember how we've looked at cutting down gradually on an unhealthy food you habitually consume or crave:

targets for cutting down on sugar and sweeteners

WEEK 1	Halve intake.
WEEK 2	Halve intake again.
WEEK 3	Have the smallest amounts possible once a day.
WEEK 4	Replace sugar with honey or blackstrap molasses or organic raw cane sugar if you must have it!

I can't think of anything further from nature than artificial sweeteners, so obviously these don't play a part in my healthy-eating plan. However, if you find it really difficult to give up sugar or sweeteners you can buy pure, organic, raw cane sugar in most stores now – if you must! I would rather see you eating a little of that than chemical-ridden artificial sweeteners.

the 3 's's: salt

Salt was so prized and valued for hundreds of years that wars were fought over it, people were paid in salt and we even named our monthly wage after it: 'salary'. It's vital for our metabolism and electrolyte balance and without it we would certainly die.

But we only need about 5–6 grams (about $\frac{1}{6}$–$\frac{1}{5}$ ounce, around a teaspoon) a day, and most of us are consuming double that amount every day. Excess sodium (salt is sodium chloride) increases blood pressure, is linked to coronary heart disease and strokes, and even to osteoporosis and stomach cancer.

The pressure group Consensus Action on Salt and Health, a collection of doctors and chefs, recently called for food manufacturers to drastically reduce the amount of 'hidden' salt in our foods, particularly in low-calorie processed foods, which can contain twice as much salt as the so-called 'unhealthy' full-fat version. The trouble is, every time fat is taken out of a meal, something has to be put in to make it tasty – and that something is usually salt!

Adding salt to our food accounts for 15–20 per cent of the salt we consume on a daily basis. Professor Graham MacGregor of St George's Hospital, Tooting, a leading expert on the relationship between salt and disease, says that just reducing salt intake to 6 grams a day could improve the health of 20,000–30,000 people a year and greatly reduce the number of deaths caused by heart disease. 'Many processed meat products, for example cheap sausages, are made from large amounts of fat, which on its own is completely inedible. To make them tasty, very large amounts of salt are added,' he says. He also warns that salt is hidden in many of the convenience foods we buy, in tins of baked beans, sweets and biscuits, bacon, even bread and cereals: 'Cornflakes contain the same amount of salt as seawater and even biscuits and manufactured cakes and puddings have the same amount of salt as potato crisps.'

Too much sodium in a diet encourages the cells to hang on to water for dear life: hence bloating and water retention. Just tick the foods on the list below that you eat regularly. Give them up for a couple of weeks, and look out for an improvement. Symptoms like bloating and water retention usually disappear quite quickly if you reduce salt intake and drink more water.

salt: worst offenders list

- Bacon (1 gram a rasher!)
- Smoked or Cured Meat like Ham
- Baked Beans (2.5 grams of salt per serving of 210 grams!)
- Margarine
- Hard Cheese like Cheddar
- Breakfast Cereals
- Biscuits
- Pizza
- Potato Crisps
- Ready Meals
- Sausages
- Smoked Fish (Just 50 grams of smoked salmon contain more than 3.75 grams of salt!)
- Tinned Soups
- Tomato Ketchup
- White Bread (One sandwich contains half the recommended daily intake in just the bread, without the filling!)

The Weekend Plan will automatically reduce your sodium intake by as much as 80–85 per cent, because the diet consists of natural fruits, vegetables and grains. You will still consume the RDA for sodium, but in an organic, absorbable form. Remember, green vegetables are full of organic sodium.

> **! TOP TIPS** FOR REDUCING SALT INTAKE
>
> Stop adding salt to your cooking.
> Stop adding salt to your food without tasting it first!
> Use other herbs and spices to add flavour, such as sea vegetables.
> Cut right down on tinned, pickled or smoked foods.
> Cut right down on ready-made meals, especially low-fat ones.
> Read the labels very carefully and look for the sodium content.
> Remember that the recommended intake is just 5–6 grams a day, which equals one teaspoon only.
> Within 2–6 weeks you won't want it any more.

the 3 's's: stimulants

alcohol

Alcohol is not, strictly speaking, a stimulant as it *depresses* the nervous system. But it does *stimulate* the liver and, as you will read later, the liver needs a good rest for 48 hours so an alcohol ban is essential during the Weekend, I'm afraid.

Alcohol is very dehydrating – remember, it's a diuretic. Just think of that thumping headache the morning after the night before. That's dehydration caused by water pouring away from important organs, such as your brain, to go and deal with your overworked kidneys.

Finally, bear in mind that alcohol turns to *sugar* and is stored by the body as *fat*. It has no other nutritional use at all, apart from making us feel relaxed and happy. Red wine is my poison, and I justify it by acknowledging that it's rich in antioxidants and has been linked to the low figures for heart disease in France! *But*, because I have such a clean body 80–90 per cent of the time, more than one glass an evening affects me quite badly. As with everything, moderation has become the name of the game, even when it comes to my favourite drink.

If you're an 'every-single-night' drinker, than cut down gradually before the Weekend, or you'll feel miserable for the whole time. Have a glass of wine or beer once or twice a week leading up to the Plan – it won't hurt. But if you can go for an extended alcohol-free period, so much the better.

> ! **TOP TIP** TO AVOID ALCOHOL-INDUCED DEHYDRATION
>
> Drink water! The average body needs approximately 4–5 molecules of water for every molecule of alcohol drunk to help remove it from the body. So drinking one glass of water for every glass of booze you drink should help your dehydration levels.

coffee

Caffeine is the most active stimulant for the nervous system. In excess it can cause insomnia, digestive problems, bowel problems, and can even harm the heart. It's a very strong diuretic, is dehydrating and, in large quantities, really dries those cells out. A gynaecologist recently told me that for a patient suffering from an unstable bladder drinking coffee (or alcohol) is so irritating that it has the same effect on the bladder as raking it with cactus spikes!

Coffee also stimulates the adrenals (little hat-shaped glands that sit on the tip of the kidneys) to produce more adrenaline, which gives the body a surge in energy for 'fight or flight'. The trouble is, if you constantly put your body into fight-or-flight mechanism, it's a bit like the boy who cried wolf too many times. The glands can't respond when needed – they've become too exhausted to produce any more adrenaline. Interestingly, the more toxins, pollutants and poor nutrition you put into your body, the more lethargic and ratty you feel, and the more you need caffeine and other stimulants to help you feel normal again. And so the cycle goes on: fluctuating blood-sugar levels followed by exhausted adrenals.

But, in moderation, coffee is a wonderful pick-me-up and my favourite stimulant. At least once a year, I give it up for three weeks and drink green tea instead, and then I definitely feel more alert in the morning and more chilled throughout the day. I do, however, usually go back to my one cup a day because I just love the whole café lifestyle that has sprung up on every high street all over the world. If at all possible, try doing without coffee completely for the Weekend and for two– three weeks after that, just to see how you feel. Organic green tea is a good alternative as it contains a tiny amount of caffeine but also an abundance of antioxidants, so the good outweighs the bad. And if you really can't function without coffee, make it just one cup of *organic* a day.

tea

Tea, on the other hand, has been getting some good press recently. It's been discovered that Britain's favourite beverage is full of antioxidants – powerful substances that help protect us from disease. Antioxidants, such as vitamins A (as beta-carotene), C and E and the mineral selenium, also neutralize any damaging free-radical molecules that may invade us, such as pollutants and toxins. So a cuppa may have some health benefits. Tea also contains theanine, which increases levels of dopamine, a 'feel-good' brain chemical, which relaxes us and makes us feel happy.

But despite those merits tea is still a diuretic, still dehydrating and still challenging to the body, especially if it's full of milk and sugar. You can get those precious antioxidants from a healthier source. So if you can't live without tea, for the sake of your soon-to-be-spring-cleaned cells reduce the number of cups you drink to a minimum and buy the purest, best leaf variety you can find. Better still, try one of the many herbal teas around. There are many choices ranging from peppermint, which calms the digestion, to camomile, which calms the mind and induces a good night's rest!

dairy products

A dairy product is anything that comes from a cow, and cow's milk is one of the most common causes of food intolerance. In fact, dairy intolerance is now one of the main food intolerances in the UK. If you suffered as a child from chronic ear infections, tonsillitis, eczema or asthma you could well be sensitive to the proteins and sugars contained in milk. Lactose and milk casein are the two usual offenders. Cow's milk is also very mucus-forming and has long been associated with chronic catarrh, sinusitis, and hay fever.

Professor Anthony Frew is an acknowledged expert in allergy and respiratory medicine at Southampton Hospital. He says that many people see considerable improvements in common conditions such as asthma, eczema, catarrh and digestive problems when they give up cow's milk and replace it with an alternative such as goat's milk. With my own clients, I'd say that figure is as high as three-quarters. Although goat's milk and cheese may well play a part in your regime after the Weekend, they're still animal products, so won't be included in the suggestions for the 48-Hour Plan.

dairy facts

Milk and cheese are hard to digest. Many nutritionists believe that cow's milk is *meant for calves*, and that human babies lose the enzyme to digest milk once breastfeeding is over, or by the age of two.

Milk and cheese can cause excessive amounts of mucus in the intestines so nutrients can't be properly absorbed.

Chronic catarrh usually clears up when dairy produce is avoided.

Cows are fed hormones and antibiotics and these are passed on to you in the milk.

The UK and the US drink more milk than probably any other country, yet we have the highest rates of osteoporosis!

Alternatives such as green vegetables and goat's milk can provide as much calcium, if not more!

Again, if you feel well on dairy produce and don't suffer from any ear, nose, chest or skin problems, then just eliminate it for the duration of the 48-Hour Plan. It doesn't need to be for life. But see how you feel when you've taken it out of your daily diet for a few days, before making any long-term decision. The following *must* be avoided over the Weekend:

dairy products

Milk   Cottage Cheese
Butter   Evaporated or Condensed
Margarine   Milk
Buttermilk   Ice Cream
Cheese   Milk Chocolate

YOGURT

Yogurt from cow's milk is the one dairy product that's an exception. It's a fermented product, and the B-vitamins that the yogurt bacteria manufacture in your gut will help you absorb calcium from all the other healthy sources you'll find in the next chapter. But make sure it's organic, plain and 'live'. (If you're going to cut out all dairy produce, then consider goat's or sheep's milk yogurt.)

wheat

It's one of the largest crops grown by humans, with evidence for its cultivation going back as far as 10,000 years. So why are we giving up wheat for the Weekend? Undoubtedly, if it's wholegrain wheat, it's a good source of complex carbohydrate (better for those sugar levels) and gives the body a healthy amount of vitamins B and E, and important minerals.

But wheat is very 'challenging' to the digestion and acid-forming, and is blamed for more digestive and bowel problems than any other food. Most of the bread and pasta on supermarket shelves nowadays tends to be poor quality, full of sugar, salt and additives. If you need proof of how many additives a cheap loaf contains, just see how many days a pre-packed loaf of sliced bread bought in the UK or the US lasts compared to a freshly baked baguette that goes stale in a matter of hours!

gluten

The other reason why so many people suffer from wheat intolerance, in the form of digestive problems such as Irritable Bowel Syndrome (IBS) and the lesser bloating, is because of the gluten. Two insoluble proteins in glutenous grains, called gliadins and glutenins, produce gluten when the flour is kneaded with water. Gluten's elastic properties make the production of bread possible. But it's the gliadin part of the mixture that appears to cause gluten intolerance – irritating the lining of the colon in a great many people. Protein in wheat is made up of as much as 55 per cent gliadin, in rye 40 per cent, and in oats just 15 per cent. *Rice and maize contain none at all.*

Wheat flour mixed with water turns into a spongy, chewing-gum-like material that literally sticks to anything. So you can imagine what it does to the inside of your intestines if the bread or pasta has not been digested properly or the intestines are dehydrated. The gluten will coat the wall of the colon, upset the beneficial bowel bacteria flora, and prevent proper absorption. Even if you are not gluten intolerant, this could, and often does, lead to constipation, discomfort, putrid bacteria, bloating and lethargy.

A healthy digestion can cope with wheaten foods such as bread, but when the system has been weakened by a long-term diet of challenging foods, difficult-to-digest substances such as gluten can build up even more problems in the gut. My personal take on this is that a truly hydrated body will not have a problem with bread, if it's of good quality and is chewed very, very well. But if the body is already stressed and 'dry' after a lifetime of poor nutrition, and bread is eaten every single day then there is a significant likelihood that, eventually, wheat intolerance will develop. According to Allergy UK, a medical charity that helps allergy-sufferers, only around 2 per cent of the UK population suffer from genuine food *allergies*; but, when it comes to wheat *intolerance*, that figure is considerably higher. 'Judging by the number of people contacting us on a daily basis,' says Chief Executive Muriel Simmonds, 'I believe 20–25 per cent of the UK is intolerant to wheat.' And if my own clients are anything to go by, I think Muriel is spot on!

For the duration of the Plan, whether you think you are wheat tolerant or intolerant, anything containing wheat (even pasta) is being taken off the menu to give your digestion a rest. And if you wake up in the night dreaming of and lusting after hot, buttered toast then you will know you probably *are* harbouring an intolerance and your body really needs this break!

animal products: meat, fish and eggs

Animal protein is full of nutrients that are absolutely essential for cell and tissue health, for body growth and repair. But animal protein takes considerable effort for the body to digest and break it down. If it's not properly broken down, the digestion can become sluggish and toxic. Meat products (sausages, pies and so on) in particular are very acid-forming and encourage the growth of unfriendly bacteria, especially if not digested properly.

1. It can take the body literally days – instead of just 24 hours with less challenging foods – to get a thick juicy steak digested and through the system from mouth to anus. As the putrid waste makes its way slowly through the intestines, it can put a heavy burden on the body's cleansing ability.

2. As we're constantly being told, a diet high in saturated fat from foods such as bacon, sausages and other processed meats can lead to higher cholesterol levels.

3. As with milk, unless they've been organically raised, the animals may have been fed hormones and antibiotics and may have eaten grass contaminated by pesticides, and these will be passed on to you in the meat.

4. *But*, although acid-forming, chicken is less challenging and fish and eggs are extremely good for you. Especially if the fish is oily (full of EFAs) and the eggs haven't been fried.

Before and after the Weekend, you can have a juicy red steak or one of the more 'challenging' meats very occasionally (such as once a month!) if you simply can't do without them. But concentrate on fish, chicken and eggs for the animal products in your diet. As oily fish is the most beneficial, you can have this three to four times a week, and chicken and eggs two or three times a week.

All animal proteins are being taken off the menu for the three days of the Plan because we want to give the digestion a weekend off. You'll get all the protein you need from nuts and seeds and other tasty snacks. In the meantime, try and:

cut down on meat, fish and animal
products in this order of priority
(The worst offenders are at the top of
the list.)

Meat Products such as Pies,   Poultry
    Sausages and Bacon   Game
Offal   Eggs
Pork   White Fish
Beef   Oily Fish
Lamb

potatoes (and aubergines, tomatoes, courgettes and peppers if you suffer from rheumatoid arthritis)

Potatoes *are* on the eliminate list. Much like wheat, they require an enormous amount of water for the intestines to break them down and assimilate them, because they're so high in starch. Although they're a very nutritious carbohydrate, which will be back on the menu after the Weekend, for the duration of the Plan they're just too challenging.

For anyone who suffers from blood-sugar problems, potatoes should only be an occasional treat. Foods such as potatoes release their sugar and starch contents very fast, which can push up glucose levels in the blood too high and too quickly, triggering fatigue and sometimes inflammation.

Which brings us on to the final reason to avoid potatoes and some of their relatives, for at least the duration of the Plan. Potatoes, tomatoes, aubergines, courgettes and peppers all contain a substance called solanine (the words comes from the Latin for nightshade). It's well known that people suffering from rheumatoid arthritis or other joint inflammation often have a dramatic reduction in pain when they avoid any foods from the nightshade family. Whether it's the solanine or the acidity of these foods that's the trigger remains to be seen. But, for anyone in pain, it's certainly worth excluding the nightshade family for just three days. For the rest of us, it's the humble potato that finishes the list of foods we should be eliminating during the 48-Hour Plan.

If you're thinking, What on earth does she expect me to eat then, please don't worry. There are plenty of alternatives in the next chapter. *And it's only for 48 hours, so keep reading — it'll be worth it, I promise!*

5. A for **Alternatives**

here they are, the plan alternatives:

2 Litres of Water a Day	Seeds
Fruit	Grains
Vegetables	Pulses
Nuts	Soya and Tofu

Does it look like a bit of a dull list? But, if you have a quick look at the recipe suggestions in chapter 17, you'll see that it isn't at all dull. There's plenty of choice for the food-and-drink routes you might want to take over the 48 Hours.

Depending on the season you pick for your detox and on your previous eating and drinking habits, some of you will accomplish a huge cleanse simply by drinking more water and cutting out wheat, the 3 'S's and animal produce. And that may well be enough. Others will find that a weekend of 'liquid only' meals, such as puréed soups and smoothies (*not* booze!), will have more of an impact. And some of you may decide that eating brown rice and steamed vegetables only will give you a really good spring clean.

Read through this section, and the meal suggestions in

chapter 17, before you make a decision. And when the time comes – taking into account the time of year – just listen to your body and see what it tells you it needs. I'm not talking about unhealthy cravings here – those are to be resisted – but about knowing instinctively which nutrients your body requires. This is something that often happens when you start drinking more water and becoming less toxic. Animals do it automatically. Some pregnant women also develop that intuition – it's not unusual for expectant mothers to feel passionate about foods such as beetroot (high in iron, potassium and folic acid, essential for a healthy foetus). When you're re-hydrated and enjoying perfect cellular balance you too will be much more in tune with what you need in the way of extra vitamins and minerals. So listen to your body! *As long as that food is included in this chapter!*

You can eat as much as you like of the suggested foods (especially the vegetables). And if you don't feel like eating anything for a day or so, that's also fine (as long as you are drinking your daily 2 litres of water). The founder of the College of Natural Nutrition, Barbara Wren, once said to me, 'Give yourself permission *not* to eat', and it's something I've never forgotten and abide by to this day. We all feel we have to eat our three square meals a day, but sometimes we don't need all three meals. We often eat out of habit, boredom or greed. On the other hand, some of us need to eat small snacks *five* times a day, or are doing so on medical advice. If that suits you better, that's fine as well. It's your body and your journey – just tune in to it.

The only thing that's cast in stone is the Alternatives list of foods, which will help cleanse and fortify you. By eating and drinking the foods with the most nutrients, energy and life in them, you'll experience better nutrition and greater vitality. So the

Weekend diet will be composed of as much 'plant' food as possible: fresh vegetables and fruit, seeds and nuts, pulses and grains.

fruit

We all know about the government's guidelines of eating 5 portions of fruit and veg a day, but *why* is fruit so important for our health?

Just look at these benefits:

fruit plus points

1. A life-bearing food: Fruit is rather clever because it carries the seeds for the next generation of trees and plants within it. It's like a big womb protecting and feeding the seeds and embryo inside it! I bet you never thought of fruit like that before! (Technically, aubergines, marrows, cucumbers and courgettes are all *fruits* because they contain the seeds of the plant. I still haven't quite worked out why the strawberry is the only fruit with its seeds on the *outside*.)

2. Aids the elimination process: Fruit helps to move excess sodium and toxins out of the cells and out of the body.

3. A balancing act: Because most fruit is alkaline, it helps prevent the body's pH from being too acidic. Also fruit is an excellent source of potassium, magnesium, calcium and sodium in the right balance and in a form the body can absorb and use. Perfect for the electrolyte balance!

4. High water content: Fruit is 70–90 per cent water, very useful for rehydrating the body.

5. High sugar content: Fruit is made up of 25–55 per cent simple *healthy* sugars, including fructose.

6. Loads of immunity-boosting vitamins, including A and C, a few Bs and E in the seeds.

7. Low in fat and high in fibre – what more could your body ask for?

SOME STARS

Papaya: Helps move debris out of the intestines.

Grapefruit: Cleans the intestinal tract and stimulates the bowel.

Pineapple: High in bromelain, an enzyme needed by the stomach for digesting, and high in vitamin C and potassium.

Melons: Have high magnesium levels, especially in the seeds.

Watermelons: A natural diuretic for flushing the kidneys, and the seeds are packed with EFAs.

Berries: Full of antioxidants. *Strawberries* are one of the most vitamin- and mineral-packed fruits you can eat, higher in vitamin C, pound for pound, than oranges.

But eating some fruits may have drawbacks for people with certain conditions. Look at the list below, and if in any doubt consult an expert.

fruit negatives

1. If you suffer from Candida or Candida symptoms such as thrush, ALL FRUIT can worsen your condition.

2. Some fruits can be hard on the digestion and cause problems for people with sensitive digestive systems. CITRUS FRUITS, such as ORANGES, TANGERINES and GRAPEFRUITS can be too acidic. (But LEMONS turn alkaline in the body and are a fantastic source of vitamin C – so they're an absolute must for everyone.)

3. Eating too many of the fruits that are very high in sugar, such as BANANAS, MELONS and GRAPES, can also affect people with blood-sugar problems.

4. SOFT FRUITS such as STRAWBERRIES and RASPBERRIES can cause aggravation for cystitis sufferers.

dried fruit

Dried fruit is a wonderful source of vitamins and minerals — dried apricots and figs are particularly high in potassium, which is very important for that electrolyte balance (and they're also a fantastic help if you need help to go to the loo). But dried fruit is very high in natural sugar. Although it's an excellent substitute for anyone missing their sugar fix, it can be fattening, challenging and cause digestion problems such as diarrhoea and flatulence if eaten in excess! So easy does it.

shopping list

Bearing in mind the plus and minus points, make up your own shopping list of fruits that will suit you and that you like. And remember: *wherever possible try and buy locally grown, seasonal fruit.* And make it organic (chapter 7 has more on why).

One final downer — I have put BANANAS on the NO list, just for the three days, as they're very starchy, play havoc with some people's insulin levels and take a lot of digesting. For the duration of the Plan, or longer, leave them out, unless you're a 12-stone man training for a marathon.

vegetables

The word vegetable comes from the Latin for to enliven or animate. So if we want to be lively and animated we need to eat lots of vegetables! Just as our red blood cells are rich in iron, the plants' equivalent of blood, chlorophyll, is rich in magnesium and other minerals that play such an important role in giving us optimum health. And because the sun produces the chlorophyll in plants, every time we eat our veg we're eating some of the sun's energy!

vegetables plus points

1. Packed full of vitamins and minerals. Vegetables are crammed with immunity-boosting, disease-fighting vitamins and minerals such as vitamin C, folic acid (from the Latin word for leaf) and selenium. Green veg are fantastically rich in nutrients, but orange, red and yellow vegetables (such as carrots and peppers) are high in beta-carotene, which produces vitamin A in our body – essential for healthy eyes, skin and tissues.

2. Cruciferous vegetables – plants that have flower petals in the shape of a cross – such as broccoli, Brussels sprouts, cabbage, kale and cauliflower, have been found by researchers to be rich in anti-cancer properties and glucosinolates – nutrients that really help the liver detox and unload.

3. Help the electrolyte balance. Dark green vegetables, such as spinach, broccoli, chard, kale, lettuce, savoy cabbage and watercress, contain high levels of the essential minerals calcium, magnesium, sodium and potassium, and in the right proportions: four times as much potassium and magnesium as sodium and calcium.

4. Very low-fat food with a good balance of carbohydrate and protein. And it's *good-quality protein* – veg is 25 per cent protein, similar to pulses, and quite enough to keep you going over the three days!

5. Full of fibre: Assist bowel movements and bowel flora. And vegetables help *clean the gut*: when eaten raw, they give the gut walls a good wipe. Steamed veg will do the job just as well.

6. Cleanse toxins from the body: A diet rich in vegetables will encourage toxicity out of the organs and tissues because the high potassium levels promote the removal of excess sodium and acidity from the body.

SOME OTHER STARS

Cabbage: Has glutamine in large quantities, which restores the digestive track.

Beetroot: Full of natural chlorine, which is a wonderful cleanser for the liver, kidneys and gall bladder.

Cucumber: Packed with silicon and sulphur for strong skin, nails and hair.

Celery: Has high levels of *organic* sodium (not table salt), which helps with elimination.

Shitake mushrooms: Boost immunity, and contain essential amino acids, making them an excellent source of protein. (They are fungi, but widely considered as the 'protein king' of veg.)

Need any more convincing why they will play such an important role during the Weekend?

seeds

Seeds are the best of the life-giving foods: they contain the embryo of a new plant or tree so all the nutrients needed to produce that huge plant or tree are present. Because they have the potential for new life, seeds are packed full of energy: don't dismiss them as just for the birds! (Anyway, when did you last see a fat, sluggish garden bird?)

seeds plus points

1. Full of Essential Fatty Acids.
2. High levels of protein. (Pumpkin seeds are over 24 per cent protein, sunflower seeds 22 per cent.)
3. Vitamin- and mineral-packed.
4. Can be eaten raw, cooked, blended or sprouted.
5. Keep blood-sugar levels even.
6. Filling, healthy snacks.

seeds for the weekend

Pumpkin seeds: Very high in zinc (which is used to treat and help prevent prostate problems) and rich in iron, calcium, phosphorus and niacin.
Sunflower seeds: Very high in potassium.
Sesame seeds: An excellent protein addition to grains such as rice, as they're rich in the amino acids that grains lack. Also high in zinc and calcium.

nuts

There are 300 types of nuts, and most of them are the fruit or seed that follows the flowering of a plant or tree. Nuts are one of nature's richest foods; they contain a good-quality protein and an even higher level of healthy fats than seeds. They're also rich in vitamins and minerals because they too provide the next generation of a plant. Because nuts are high in fat, many people avoid them when trying to lose weight. But they contain *unsaturated* fat and essential fatty acids (which we'll explore in detail in chapter 14). Because of those precious oils, shelled nuts can easily turn rancid if not stored in cool, dry places away from air. (This also applies to seeds.) I keep all of mine mixed together in an airtight container in the fridge.

Roasted or salted nuts are not included in the Weekend Plan, but all the following nuts are and, as suggested above, you can toast them yourself without adding any salt or fat.

the best nuts for the weekend: the shopping list

Almonds: Best all-round nuts as their fat content is less than most other nuts; high in protein (nine almonds provide the full daily protein requirement for an adult male!), EFAs, vitamins E and some Bs. Also high calcium levels.

Brazil nuts: More fat than almonds, but very high in selenium, which is good for protecting immunity and helping the liver detox.

Hazelnuts: Higher in Vitamin E, good for the skin.

Peanuts: Not a true nut, more a legume or pulse, which is why it has the word pea in its name! Peanuts are an excellent source of protein, but aren't the easiest nuts to digest.

Walnuts: Look a bit like a brain when they are out of their shell, and that's exactly what they're good for – the brain!

grains

Grains are the seeds of various grasses and cereals (such as wheat and barley). As seeds, grains are also full of life, and some of them, *but not all*, need to be seriously considered for their nutritional value and their cleansing ability this Weekend. Have a look at the menus in chapter 17 to see which grains you haven't tried before that you might want to experiment with before the Weekend.

But, remember, you'll be cutting out wheat, at least for the Plan. So start thinking about taking wheat-based bread out of your diet. If you're used to eating sandwiches every day, there are plenty of wheat-free breads on sale now in major supermarkets and health shops. And some of them taste as good as the 'real thing'. You'll be amazed at the difference if you start replacing the wheat in bread or pasta with gentler grains such as brown basmati rice. See how well you feel.

There are plenty of alternatives to wheat, but they should be considered in order of preference, millet being the most alkaline and rye being the most acidic. The millet end of the list is the best, and the rye end is the most challenging and not the most appropriate for a cleanse:

grain alternatives

Millet
Rice
Quinoa
Barley
Corn
Oats
Rye

millet

No, not something you feed to the parrot, but *numero uno* on the best-of-the-grains chart. Millet has been used in China for thousands of years. It consists of small round grains which can be ground into flour and made into a porridge-like food or even bread.

Millet is *very* gentle on the system and full of magnesium, potassium and iron, as well as being very high in protein and low in starch. It's also a non-glutenous grain and the most alkaline and as such is the least congesting in the digestive system. It's ideal for a detox, as it's so warming and soothing, and it's suitable for people with digestive problems; however it's not the easiest food to turn into a tasty meal. But don't worry – check out the recipe in chapter 17.

rice

This is the second most consumed grain in the world after wheat, and my favourite. But it has to be *brown* rice. White rice has little left of the B vitamins, the healthiest part of the grain has been refined away, and it has usually been bleached, cleaned, pearled (polished with talc), oiled and coated! It may be more digestible than wheat but there is very little nutrition in it.

Wholegrain or *brown rice*, on the other hand, is packed full of vitamin B (wonderful for the nervous system) and has the added bonus of containing an oil called gamma-oryzanol, which helps heal the digestive gut. Best of all, brown rice is one of the most efficient and easily available colon-cleansers known to man! Brown rice acts just like a broom in your intestines, sweeping away all manner of stuff that has got stuck to the sides over the years. Eating brown rice is also very helpful to the liver while it's detoxing, because it gives this important organ all the minerals and vitamins it needs to do a better job.

Short-grain organic brown rice is the best, but personally I find it a bit too starchy, and much prefer organic basmati brown rice, which is much lighter and easier to cook. Try both and see what you think.

quinoa

Quinoa (pronounced keen-waa) is a traditional native plant from the Andes, dating back to the time of the Incas. It has been hailed as the 'mother grain' because of its importance in the region's diet. Nutritionally compared to rice, it's even higher in protein, very high in calcium and magnesium and generous in its iron levels. Quinoa contains all the essential amino acids, making it a complete-protein food, and it's very easily digestible – but it's a little bland, I find, unless you jazz it up.

barley

There's evidence for the use of barley as far back as 6000 BC. But now it's used mainly in animal feed or beer and whisky. It's quite a glutenous grain, but in cereal or bread form is certainly much better for your gut than wheat. It can also be added to soups and stews to bulk them up.

corn or maize

Maize is relatively high in vitamins and minerals, especially vitamin A. Fresh corn is also very high in vitamin C and is, in fact, the main source of manufactured vitamin C in the US.

Before the corn grains mature the maize is harvested as sweetcorn. Once matured the corn is used to make tortillas, polenta, popcorn, cornflakes and cornflour. While there is no place for popcorn or cornflakes during the Plan, there is definitely one for polenta, as you will see in the recipes chapter. If you're craving carbohydrate and don't like brown rice, this isn't a bad substitute.

oats

These are a big favourite in Scotland, which has the perfect climate to grow oats! The grains can be crushed and split and made into flour for foods such as oatcakes and oatmeal. But oats are probably best known for their use as a breakfast dish – in the form of porridge – and for their ability to lower cholesterol.

Oatcakes and porridge are good replacements while you're trying to wean yourself off wheat, but don't play a big part in the Weekend Plan because they can be quite acid-forming (and often contain hidden salt and sugar). However, if you decide to do the Plan in the middle of a freezing winter, porridge *is* a great start to the day — without the cream and sugar! (Use a little rice- or soya-milk instead, and check the packaging for hidden extras!)

rye

Pumpernickel and other rye breads and crispbreads are very popular in Scandinavia and Germany. Rye flour contains very little gluten, but it does make the bread very dense and heavy. It's also the most acidic of the grains, after wheat, so doesn't really figure during the Plan.

However, rye is quite useful as a wheat substitute during your build-up, and post Plan, as it converts to sugar very slowly in the body, which means your insulin levels won't go flying all over the place. Try and buy organic brands, as some dark 'rye' breads are made of wheat flour with only a little rye and dye added to darken them!

I'm not a big fan of crispbreads because they so often have unacceptably high levels of sodium and other substances added. But I do appreciate they have a very useful role to play, and if you like them just make sure you get the very best you can find! (You might like to try rice cakes as an alternative but, again, make sure they're not full of salt.)

pulses

A pulse is an edible, ripe, dried seed of a legume – vegetables that are in a special class all of their own because their seeds grow *inside* pods that appear after the plant flowers. Common pulses are:

Aduki Beans	Black-Eye Beans
Chickpeas	Lentils
Pinto Beans	Puy Lentils
Flageolet Beans	Green Peas
Kidney Beans	Peanuts

These valuable little seeds are a mixture of protein and starch, low in fat and high in fibre. For vegetarians and for the duration of the Plan, pulses are a good source of protein – but they're what's called an 'incomplete' protein because they don't have all eight of the essential amino acids that the body needs. To make them complete, pulses need to be eaten with grains: the best example is baked beans on toast! Sadly, that particular favourite is not on the Weekend menu, but there are other tasty alternatives such as hummus accompanying rice. Aduki beans are the most detoxifying of the pulses. In Chinese medicine they are the best bean for tackling water retention and are good for the spleen. (There's an aduki bean salad suggestion in chapter 17.)

One of the main problems with eating pulses is wind! This is largely caused by the sugars (oligosaccharides) in the beans fermenting away in the lower intestines. If the beans are soaked overnight and then rinsed, you will get rid of most of the sugars and the resultant bloating.

soya and tofu

The soya bean – high in protein and low in fat – is also a pulse and, with the peanut, is one of the most complete proteins of the legume family. Soya beans also contain compounds called phytoestrogens – natural plant oestrogens, which help women's bodies maintain hormonal balance as their oestrogen levels fluctuate. In fact, unwelcome menopausal symptoms are practically unheard of in Japan, where they eat a lot of soya. You can certainly add soya beans to any dishes you're preparing during the detox.

Tofu is made from soya beans by fermenting them. The end result is a block of tofu or silken tofu, which can be cubed and added to salads and stir-fries or blended into dressings. Although it looks a bit like a slab of rubber, tofu is very useful in cooking, as it's a good meat substitute and takes on the flavours of any foods cooked with it.

Tofu is more and more visible on our supermarket shelves in the guise of meat-free sausages, rissoles, burgers and other snacks. These are likely to be high in salt and additives, unless you buy an organic brand, so check the ingredients carefully.

Tofu products and soya milk can also be quite mucus-forming, so they don't play a huge part in the detox Plan. However, for anyone who simply can't live without meat, milk or mayonnaise during the Weekend, or post-Plan, a little tofu and soya milk may be included.

So, there are all your Alternatives. Have a look at the recipes chapter to reassure yourself that this isn't going to be a weekend of just eating rabbit food and that there are lots of appetizing options when it comes to healthy eating.

In the next chapter, we look at the lymphatic system and

how it can help us speed up the whole cleansing process. You'll also discover some new and interesting techniques to try out which will benefit your long-term health as well as helping your detox along.

6. L for **Lymph**

The lymphatic system is like the guttering of the body. From all over it collects and takes away the cells' rubbish. This debris is filtered by the lymph nodes for infectious invaders and then dumped into the bloodstream to circulate to the liver, where it's further broken down and eliminated. The lymphatic system is a secondary circulatory system, running alongside the blood but, unlike blood, it has no pump of its own and relies on a little bit of help to get it going. It's full of lymph, a pale yellow, watery fluid that is very similar to blood plasma in composition. Every time we breathe or move we are helping 3 litres (over 5 pints) of lymph to circulate through the lymphatic system via the nodes and out into the blood.

Hundreds of lymph nodes are dotted all over the body. They're oval or bean-shaped and can be as small as a pinhead or up to the size of a large kidney bean. These clever little filtering plants prevent any infection or foreign particle from travelling on into the bloodstream and spreading throughout the body. Lymph nodes also produce and store lymphocytes, white blood cells that fight infection by ingesting bacteria. It is the nodes that we can feel as little hard lumps when we are run down or infected – usually in the area closest to the infection.

where are my lymph nodes?

Neck
Groin
Behind the Knees
Armpits
All over the Breasts

Above the Elbow
Tonsils, Adenoids, Appendix
Small Intestine

When the lymphatic system gets blocked by an infection or overloaded by excessive toxins things can start going wrong. A congested lymph node won't drain properly, the system's circulation slows down and the cells don't get enough nourishment or protection. Swollen glands, aches and pains, a sore throat, a temperature and itchy skin are all signs of being run down and having toxicity or a virus stuck in the cells and lymph. Water retention is also a sign of blocked lymph. The tissues will react according to where the lymph is blocked in the body. For example, if the lymph nodes in the head and neck are congested, your complexion can look dull and you may be holding more water than usual around your chin.

Salon treatments such as Manual Lymphatic Drainage can really help a sluggish lymphatic system, but you can give it a boost yourself at home on a daily basis.

how to get lymph moving:

Skin-Brushing.
Alternate Hot and Cold Water in the Shower.
Exercise Daily.
Give Yourself Regular Massage.

skin-brushing

The skin is our largest organ and, just like the kidneys, liver and colon, it's an eliminating organ that gets rid of more than half a kilo (one lb) of waste and toxins each and every day. If the skin gets choked up by millions of dead cells and clogged pores, toxins and impurities will stay in the body, and the other eliminating organs will have to work harder to clear the waste.

This is a really simple, quick and effective technique that'll help your skin eliminate that waste. Skin-brushing can be done before your shower or bath each day – and definitely over the Weekend, when you'll have more time. It only takes 10 minutes, but you can do it in five when you're in a real hurry.

benefits of daily skin-brushing

Boosts blood circulation.
Stimulates the lymph.
Helps fight cellulite.
Softens skin.
Helps prevent skin infections and irritations.
Freshens body.
Rejuvenates.

First, if you haven't already done so, buy a body brush. Make sure it's from a natural source and not plastic. (But don't go for 'natural bristle', because that's made from badger hair!) There are plenty on sale these days and you can usually find a reasonable one in a health shop, beauty salon or even super-market.

Before showering or bathing, on dry skin, start brushing

firmly UP TOWARDS THE HEART, starting from the soles of your feet. Work up the front of each leg to your abdomen. Brush your tummy with circular movements in a CLOCKWISE direction. Carry on brushing upwards to the bottom of your breasts. Then work all the way UP the back of your legs, past your bottom, as far as you can reach, and brushing as vigorously as feels comfortable. The bottom and thighs are good areas to concentrate on as they usually carry the most fat cells!

When you get to your upper chest and upper back, change the direction and start brushing from the neck DOWN-WARDS TOWARDS THE HEART, both front and back, always in the direction that the blood flows to the heart. Finally, brush your hands and all the way UP each arm, on the top and the underside. And don't forget to brush inside your armpit by holding your arm up and brushing DOWNWARDS.

Don't do your face, but you can give the back of your neck and your scalp a good going-over!

You should feel very energized at the end of this session. By the conclusion of the Plan, when you can see and feel the benefits of skin-brushing, you'll want to find five minutes every morning to carry on. Why not start now?

hot and cold showering

If you haven't got a body brush, or are away from home without it, here's another way to help the lymph flow and boost your immune system. Have a shower, and when you've reached the end of your ablutions turn the shower on as cold as you can stand it for 10 seconds (building up over time to 30 seconds), then turn it up to warm again for a minute or two. Repeat this three or four times, and end on cool. As the hot water warms up your skin, the blood – and therefore the lymph – rushes up to the surface of your body to keep the heat away from precious organs. As the cold water hits the surface of your skin, the blood and the lymph rush away from the surface of your skin to protect the organs. So you can see this is a really good way to get things pumping – and it's free!

> **! TOP TIP** FOR CELLULITE-BUSTING
>
> If you have a fairly high-powered shower, you might like to
> try this as a cellulite-buster. Using a hand-held shower,
> with the water pressure up as high as it'll go, concentrate
> on blasting the areas of cellulite – thighs, buttocks,
> upper arms, etc. – using a circular movement.

exercise

Exercising daily is essential if you want to get a sluggish lymphatic system going because as it doesn't have a pump of its own it relies on muscular activity to pump the lymph fluid *upwards*. It doesn't matter what you do – as long as you do it *regularly*. Gentle jogging is excellent, but does not suit all of us. Brisk walking, especially uphill, is just as good, and 10–20 minutes of this a day is all that is needed. But more is better!

rebounder

One of the best exercises for the lymph has to be jumping up and down on a rebounder – a mini trampoline – for 10 minutes a day. If you happen to have one lurking around under a bed somewhere, dig it out, put on some loud music and start bouncing. Bouncing works with the earth's natural gravity, which means that when you get to the top of a bounce for a nanosecond you're weightless, and at the bottom of the bounce gravity is increased by two or three times. This will really encourage the lymph to shift toxins, as well as halving the impact on your joints.

swimming-pool bouncing

If you don't have a rebounder there is a very good and cheap alternative: bouncing up and down in a swimming pool – or in the sea if it's warm enough. The water will bear your weight so, again, there will be no stress to the joints. Get far enough into the pool so that the water reaches your breastbone, then start jumping up and down, using the water as support. Or gently run on the spot in the water.

If you're not in the habit of taking regular exercise, start off slowly and build up your exercise routine. There are more suggestions in chapter 10, all of which will help get the lymph going.

self-massage

As well as giving you a bit of a pamper, deep-tissue massage will also help move the lymph – and it's something you can do at home with this simple version. What you'll be doing is slightly different from ordinary salon massage, in that you will be squeezing and stretching the connective tissues which are made up of fluids and fibres. This creates a cleansing, flushing effect similar to rinsing out a sponge, or stirring the water in a ditch that is clogged with algae!

This DIY version has been compiled for you by Janie Hildebrand, a deep-tissue masseuse, who I see regularly to benefit my neglected emotional senses, touch and smell! In between visits, I find the following plan very quick and easy to do straight after a shower or bath.

diy method

So that your hands glide over your skin easily, and to make it softer, use either almond oil or cold-pressed virgin olive oil, or any other oil you have in the house that suits your skin and doesn't offend your nose. They all work well as 'carrier' oils, as well as feeding your skin, and, as this Weekend is all about relaxing, you might also like to consider adding an essential oil.

CARRIER OILS

SKIN-TYPE	OIL
All	Almond
Oily & Combination	Grapeseed
Sensitive	Jojoba
Dry, Sun-Damaged	Vitamin E
All (if nothing else available)	Virgin Olive

ESSENTIAL OILS

SKIN-TYPE	OIL
All – Relaxing	Lavender
Dry & Mature Skins	Frankincense
Mature Skin	Rose
Very Dry Skin	Patchouli

Oily, Spotty Skin	Sandalwood
All – Antiseptic	Tea Tree & Eucalyptus
All	Jasmine

Have a look at the suggestions and pick your essential and carrier oils. For massages, essential oils are NOT to be used neat. Put 1–2 tablespoons of the carrier oil into a little bowl. Then add 3–6 drops of your chosen essential oil and mix it through. For repeated use you could also fill a little plastic bottle with a carrier oil and then add 5–10 drops of your essential oil; give the bottle a good shake every time.

Make sure you put plenty of the mixed oils on your hands or fingers so that these glide over your skin, much like when applying body lotion. It's amazing how quickly a dry skin will lap it up, so keep putting on more oil till you're really greased up! Don't be afraid of it. The more you put on, the easier it is to carry out the suggested movements.

Again, because we are helping the lymph move, it's important to always work in the direction of the blood flow to the heart. You work from the head DOWN and from the legs and stomach UP, just as you do with skin-brushing, but this time start with the head. You might prefer to do a massage *after* your bath or shower, when the skin is nice and warm and a little damp. You might find it best to sit on the edge of the bath, on the loo, or on a towel on the floor. Experiment and see what works for you.

HEAD

To begin with, sit up straight in a comfy but supporting chair, or on the floor with your back against something. Slowly 'shampoo' your scalp all over, using the pads of your fingers, not your nails, working the oil well into the scalp. This movement is incredibly relaxing as well as being very good for your hair. Leave the oil on while you carry on with the rest of the massage.

FACE

Warm a teaspoon of your mixed oils in your palms. Rub your hands together and then press them all over your face quickly and firmly. Using your fingertips, tap lightly and quickly all over your face, starting from the centre and working outwards: along your eyebrows, under eyes, along the cheekbones, around your mouth and along your chin. Then, using your fingers, make little circles starting at the hairline and working down round the outside of the face. As you reach the chin, gently pinch the flesh between fingers and thumbs, working from the point of the chin to the ears. Then using the index fingers and thumbs gently pinch the eyebrows, moving outwards. Massage the middle of your forehead and the temples in circular motions. With two or three of your middle fingers, start at the nose and gently sweep along the bone under the eye, moving *out* from the nose towards your ears. Do the same under the cheekbones, sweeping outwards from nose to ears. Then put your fingers under the middle of your nose and sweep downwards above the mouth, following the line of your upper lip. And, finally, put your fingers under the middle of your bottom lip and sweep upwards and out, again following the line of your lip. Finish the face by pulling on the ear lobes and give them a good massage. This will help the blood flow to your face and wake up your complexion. Lastly, rub your hands together quite fast and then place them over your face, keeping your eyes closed. Inhale the essential oils and the heat radiating from your hands.

NECK AND SHOULDERS

Very hard to do on yourself, but what you can do, with a well-oiled hand, is to pinch the flesh along the top of your shoulder blade, between the first three fingers and thumb of the opposite hand, moving up and down the entire length of each shoulder. And then, with one hand, very gently massage the back of your neck.

ARMS

Try and cup the whole of the opposite arm by placing your fingers on top and your thumb underneath. Start at the wrist and, using upward strokes, glide up the arm, pressing firmly. Repeat several times on each arm, alternating between thumb on top and thumb underneath.

FEET

In a seated position, put a foot on the opposite knee. Cradle your toes in the same-side hand, and with your opposite hand, using your knuckles only, circle all over the bottom of your foot. Squeeze the back and sides of the foot above the heel. This is where a lot of tension is held. Finish by pulling each toe firmly and briskly, making sure each one is oiled. Repeat on the other foot.

LEGS AND THIGHS

With one foot up on the side of the bath, cup your two hands around both sides of the leg, from above the anklebone, and firmly and slowly glide both hands together right up the leg and over the knee. You might have to do this several times to make sure your whole leg has been massaged. Re-oil your hands and repeat the same on your thighs as high up as you can, but this time you can use more pressure. Repeat on the other leg.

ABDOMEN AND BOTTOM

For the abdomen, just use circular movements, in a clockwise direction, as gently or as firmly as you feel comfortable with. A lot of people don't like having their tummies massaged so see how you feel. The bottom is a very difficult muscle to work on your own, so instead give it a good scrub with a loofah when you're in the shower!

And talking of showers – do resist the urge to jump in and wash off the oil. It won't take long for most of it to soak in. Don't forget that your skin is the body's largest organ and anything on it, good or bad, is absorbed into the bloodstream. So try not to wash the benefits away. Instead, wrap up warmly in an old towelling dressing gown and have a lie-down!

Practise self-massage whenever you get a chance to spend a little bit of 'me time' in the bathroom. Apart from helping your lymph, it's good to get into the habit of looking after yourself and monitoring your stress levels. Beneficial techniques such as self-massage and skin-brushing shouldn't be rationed to a once-a-year treat, so get into the habit of doing them more often from now on. You and your body deserve them!

You also deserve a rest from all the toxins that bombard us in ever-increasing amounts, and that's what we'll be looking at next. You might be surprised by the list of things that I consider to be toxic – but after thinking about it you might even add some more that I haven't considered!

7. T for **Tackling Toxins**

According to some medical experts, toxins don't exist. It depends on what you define as a toxin. Most holistic practitioners, myself included, consider toxins to be any substance that gets into the cells and causes an imbalance. This can be anything from chemicals in food to air pollution, from sugar in a fizzy drink to painkillers. Anything that we breathe in, ingest or touch could be considered toxic by our body. Anything that undermines our health or places stress on our organs – including negative thoughts and anger.

Check this list and see how many of the 'toxins' listed below are ruling your life and affecting your health. Add to that list if you think of any more. After you've read the book once through, come back to this list and put asterisks next to the stressers you would really like to live without over the Weekend – and, hopefully, for ever.

toxins

- Processed and Pre-Packaged Foods
- Snacks and Fizzy Drinks
- Fast Food and Takeaways
- Pesticides and Chemicals in Non-Organic Food
- Coffee and Tea
- Alcohol

- Sugar
- Nicotine
- Prescription Drugs
- Over-the-Counter Medicines
- 'Recreational' Drugs
- Regular Airline Travel
- Regular Tube or Metro Travel
- Regular Car Use
- Electrical Gadgets and Electromagnetic Field Emissions
- Regular TV Viewing
- Regular Computer Use
- Regular Mobile Use
- Unhealthy Relationships
- Stressful Job
- Stressful Home
- Little or no Exercise
- Little or no Fresh Air or Sunlight
- Always-on-the-go
- Don't Meditate
- Don't do Breathing Exercises
- Don't do Yoga or similar
- No Time to just sit and be
- No Time to relax
- No Time for 'me'!

processed and packaged foods

If you needed reminding of why you're giving up packaged and processed foods and drinks, consider this. One of Britain's leading authorities on food, Dr Erik Millstone, Reader in Science Policy at the University of Sussex, estimates that no fewer than 5,000 chemicals are used as additives in packaged foods and drinks in the UK today. He has calculated that an average person on today's diet consumes *6–7 kilos* of additives every year – some of them harmless flavourings, but many of them untested, and therefore considered to be potentially unsafe.

non-organic food

According to Roz Kadir, Nutritionist to the England Rugby Squad, the amount of chemical pesticides, herbicides and fungicides used on conventional crops has very worrying health implications: 'Eating non-organic produce is like taking part in a long-term experiment, swallowing something like *one gallon* of pesticides and organophosphates a year.'

Organic produce may seem comparatively expensive but, as a mother of two, Roz believes it's money well spent. 'My children are already bombarded by pollution from the environment – why add to that load and potentially risk their long-term health?'

reasons to eat organic food

It tastes better!

It's been grown or reared without artificial chemicals, pesticides and fertilizers, so it's safe, nutritious, unadulterated food.

It's environmentally friendly.

It's produced without genetically modified ingredients.

It places greater emphasis on animal welfare.

It's produced without the routine use of antibiotics and growth-promoting drugs.

It relies on a modern and scientific understanding of ecology and soil science, but it also depends on traditional methods of crop rotation to ensure soil fertility and weed and pest control.

It's natural food – just as nature intended!

I would recommend always buying the freshest and purest quality of fruit and vegetables you can afford – within reason.

But before you go out and fill your basket full of organic fruit and veg, first look at the labels and see how far the produce has travelled. In an ideal natural world, organic fruit and veg would be sold locally and in season. But that doesn't often happen. I don't see the point of buying organic apples if they've been flown all the way from New Zealand, or Spanish strawberries that have been ripening en route for three days, when the UK produces some of the best apples and strawberries in the world. Think how *you* feel after a three-day journey. The longer it takes from the farm to your fork, the fewer nutrients will be available by the time you eat that apple or strawberry; and the higher the cost of transporting that fruit to your local supermarket.

Of course, one effective way of guaranteeing the 'freshness' of produce, apart from picking your own, is to use *frozen organic* fruit and veg. It can be even more expensive, but it does mean you can buy, for example, unadulterated English berries out of season, store them at your convenience and add a few at a time to liven up a smoothie or pudding. Because the nutrients have been locked in during the freezing process, frozen organic produce is worth considering from time to time.

If you're going to juice, blend or purée any fruit or vegetable, it's even more important that it should be as free of chemicals as possible. If you're juicing a whole carrot you're extracting not only 90 per cent of the vitamins and minerals, but also 90 per cent of any pesticides. What's the point of making lovely healthy soups or juices if they're packed full of chemicals?

The compromise for the sake of your health and your purse might lie in shopping at one of the growing number of farmers' markets. Here you can buy direct from a local farmer, and know the food has been grown within a reasonable distance of where you live, even if you're in a city. The fruit and veg will be *richer in nutrients*, because it hasn't been ripened artificially during a long journey. The food should be *cheaper* because the growers have cut out the middleman. And it'll be *seasonal*, so you'll be eating what you were naturally meant to be eating at that time of year. If you find a really good farmers' market near you but the produce is *not* organic, don't get too stressed about it unless you're juicing, in which case it *should* be organic whenever possible. Small fruit and vegetable farmers don't as a rule use excessive amounts of pesticides and chemicals. Ask them. If you're not sure, wash thoroughly and peel, top and tail the produce.

If you're lucky enough to live in the country you might not even need a market as your local farmer will probably be selling fruit and veg at the bottom of his drive, or offering pick-your-own. Best of all, you might be able to grow some of your food yourself, and control exactly what goes into it.

In cities there are more and more organic supermarkets popping up that will sell all the organic produce you might need, but it'll be more expensive. You're paying for food that has been grown to the highest ethical and quality standards but, again, check the labels to see how many air miles it's done.

And, of course, there are the supermarket giants. In certain parts of the country, their organic sections are enormous, such is our demand for chemical- and pesticide-free food. The more we buy, the more competitive their prices become, so your local supermarket is also well worth checking out.

You may end up, like me, buying from two or three different sources. I appreciate that some of you won't have the time to shop around on a weekly basis, but I hope you'll be able to do so for the Plan. I buy organic vegetables and fruit – for juicing and making smoothies – from the local supermarket; and I buy as much organic produce as I can from the local farmers' market. If I can't find the organic version of an ingredient for a particular recipe I will occasionally buy non-organic, but wash it really well.

People always throw up their hands in horror at the price of organic fruit and veg but for the Weekend, as you're not buying meat, fish or ready meals, the shopping bill's still going to be less than normal.

Be aware, though, that an organic label doesn't always mean 'healthy'. An organic pizza, for example, is still full of fat, gluten and salt – however organic these are! And only *some* of the pizza's ingredients need to be organically produced for it to be allowed an organic label, so don't be conned – just because a processed food is labelled as organic, it's not necessarily good for you or great for your digestion! Read the ingredients list and use your common sense. Indigestible organic food will still add to your toxic load because it makes the colon more sluggish.

At the end of the day, if your budget allows for it, the organic fruit and veg route is the least toxic route. But if you can't afford it, or can't find what you want in an organic range, I would much rather see you eating more fruit and veg – even if it's non-organic, as long as every piece is 'topped and tailed' and washed and peeled!

coffee and tea

If coffee and tea aren't organically grown, toxic chemicals are usually used on the crop; and 'decaf' coffee is even worse, because chemicals such as methylene chloride or trichloroethylene are employed to decaffeinate the beans and leave toxic residues. If you want decaf, make sure it's been prepared by the 'water or Swiss process', which means steam distillation is used to remove the caffeine. If you can't live without your daily cup, try to drink just one cup of organic, pure coffee or tea a day. And don't forget that caffeine is hiding in many of our painkillers and soft drinks – which you'll be cutting down on or out!

alcohol

Certainly as far as your liver is concerned alcohol is a toxin. Around 95 per cent of the alcohol you consume has to be metabolized by your liver, which requires a lot of work. As far as *you* are concerned, if you're in the habit of having a drink or two every evening, it will do you the world of good to prove that you don't *need* alcohol to relax for three days. There are warning signs to suggest that someone might be on the way to becoming an alcoholic: habitually drinking alone, drinking every day, frequently skipping a proper meal in favour of a 'liquid lunch'. But if you can easily stop drinking for a week or two at a time – or at least a day or two – you have nothing to worry about.

sugar and artificial sweeteners

Sugar, as we've seen earlier, reduces immunity, is addictive and is blamed for many of our 21st-century diseases such as adult-onset diabetes. As far as toxicity goes, the millions of micro-organisms that share our space – on our skin, in our gut and everywhere around us – love sweet foods. A diet high in sugar allows them to take over and infest us with bacteria, fungi and parasites, which leads to toxicity in the cells and conditions such as Candida (a severe form of pH imbalance causing thrush and bloating) or, at worst, diabetes.

90 per cent of people who have Candida got it from excess sugars.

As far as *artificial sweeteners* are concerned, for the reasons described earlier, they don't play a part in a healthier-eating plan. We don't know enough about the chemicals used to make them, and the long-term effects of those chemicals. They have had a sufficiently bad press to be considered as toxins as far as your health is concerned, and, anyway, they don't seem to be that successful when it comes to weight loss, do they?

There are four main artificial sweeteners used in foods in the UK today – saccharin, acesulfame-K, aspartame and cyclamate – and they're used as bulk sweeteners in the majority of processed foods. Avoid them all!

nicotine

Nicotine has been described as the hardest drug to kick, and it is probably the most toxic. In its liquid form nicotine is a powerful poison: a single injection of just one drop would be absolutely lethal. It's the nicotine in cigarettes, not the smoke, that has us hooked, and many experts consider it to be even more addictive than heroin.

Smoking causes irritation, inflammation and allergies, and destroys antioxidants such as vitamin C, so the immune system overall is weakened. Cigarettes contain thousands of toxic chemicals in the smoke and tar, which we know to cause bronchitis, emphysema, cancer and many other diseases. They age our skin, make our teeth and fingers yellow and may eventually kill us!

Enough said. I know it's hard, but if you're a smoker you

know better than anyone else that this is one toxin that has to go. So use thinking about the Weekend as an opportunity to plan to give up for good. Make a date with a hypnotherapist, go to the doctor to discuss nicotine-replacement therapy (although some substitutes can be just as toxic), or join a self-help group. Start cutting down now, and by the Weekend you'll have your 'crutches' in place, or will have given up altogether. Whatever you do, don't decide to go 'cold turkey' that particular weekend. I've been there and can vouch for how addictive nicotine is, and how much you can suffer from withdrawal symptoms unless you have a nicotine substitute or some other help.

drugs: prescription, over-the-counter or recreational

Your consumption of any drugs also needs to be reduced as much as possible during your detox. All drugs, whether legal or illegal, herbal or pharmaceutical, have some toxicity and it's the liver's job to break that down and get rid of it. Your liver will really benefit from a rest this weekend, so for optimum results, give it the break it needs.

Prescribed medicines such as painkillers, sleeping pills, tranquillizers and antidepressants can be effective for suppressing pain, inflammation and troublesome emotions, and for helping us relax and sleep. But they don't always address the *reason* we're suffering in the first place. The 48-Hour Plan will, hopefully, help you look for and find the cause. I'm certainly not suggesting that you immediately throw away any prescription drugs you might need for insomnia or depression, but do discuss their use with your doctor and see if you can eventually wean yourself off or on to a herbal, more natural version, such as St John's wort. It's important to do this gradually and with medical advice, so that you don't suffer any withdrawal problems.

Similarly, if you constantly take over-the-counter treatments for symptoms like headaches, backache, constipation or indigestion, try to do without them for at least the three days, preferably longer. Your liver will really appreciate the rest. Dr Simon Ellis, Consultant Neurologist at North Staffordshire Hospital, advises that if you're taking over-the-counter pain-killers for more than seven days per month, that's excessive. Use the Weekend as an opportunity to stop relying on them.

If you habitually roll up a joint every evening to relax, or indulge in other social recreational drugs, the Weekend will give you a wonderful chance to prove to yourself that you don't need to rely on them. Despite being a 'herb', marijuana includes tetrahydrocannabinol, which gets stored in the body fat and liver, so any routine user should have at least one annual detox. Any social drug contains toxic chemicals so cut them out of your life for at least the three days.

travel

Travelling, in all its shapes or forms, seems to be making us ill and causing toxicity in our bodies. Travelling in itself shouldn't be bad for you, but the modern way of life and the conditions of modern transport can make it so. For example, the London Underground system is full of lead, asbestos and all manner of toxins, including electromagnetic waves. Crowded conditions in packed carriages are perfect for distributing germs from one person to another, and together with delays can cause stress.

If you use the car every day, you doubtless get worked up in the traffic, and are breathing in the exhaust fumes all around you. Even cyclists, who after all are exercising healthily, now wear mouth masks to protect them from the pollution in our cities, pollution that has been linked to rising figures for asthma and other bronchial conditions.

If you fly regularly you can also get stressed, suffer jet lag and catch other people's germs from the recycled cabin air. Added to that there are the exposure to ozone and radiation at high altitudes, the lack of oxygen, the pollution, the increased dehydrating effects of alcohol and the risk of DVT (deep-vein thrombosis) from the cramped conditions. Sounds hideous!

Unfortunately, commuting is a fact of daily life for many of us, and many people travel regularly by plane on business. So make a point of minimizing travel stress for the Weekend. Hopefully, the most you'll need to do is to use your car to get away from it all.

electrical goods

All electrical appliances emit electromagnetic fields (EMFs). According to Powerwatch (an independent body monitoring EMF issues), some appliances give off levels higher even than are found under the most powerful *overhead transmission line*. Alasdair Phillips, an electrical engineer and Director of Powerwatch says, 'Many scientists believe the EMFs around us, because of our increased consumption of electricity, may be damaging our health. They can weaken our immune system and encourage diseases like cancer and Alzheimer's.' Even a few minutes' use of some electrical appliances can lead to depression, headaches, mood swings, anxiety, low energy and poor concentration.

Powerwatch has expressed concern over many household items because they emit EMFs and because we use most of them, *day in*, *day out*, without knowing the long-term health implications. It's the fact that we keep these items so close to our bodies and use them for such long spells that makes the EMFs potentially harmful. Electromagnetic fields are measured in milligauss – mobile phones are at the top of the 'avoid scale', emitting a staggering 100 milligauss, while digital clocks are near the bottom, giving off only 6 milligauss. Even if the EMFs emission is that low, I still think it's worth seeing how you feel at the end of a weekend having turned everything *off*. (There are some things, like the washing machine and iron, that you might be delighted to avoid over the Weekend!)

I'm not suggesting that you stop using the appliances for any longer than the length of the Plan – unless you want to – because they can make our lives easier and more comfortable. And, anyway, you're going to be so well protected and armed in the future by your diet and lifestyle that your cells will be better able to cope with a few EMFs and toxins! (And there are tips in chapter 18 on using them more safely.)

And it isn't just the EMFs that have to be considered. The Weekend is supposed to be calming you down, allowing your nervous system to relax and your cells to regenerate. Any external 'noise' – blaring radio, shuddering washing machine – will interfere with that. Remember that we're suffering from an auditory and visual overload, so we need to shut everything off. Just for three days.

tv

TV sets emit EMFs, which may affect you, especially if you sit too close to the screen. And the visual stimulus of a TV screen excites the nervous system even if the programme is low-key. TVs also generate static electricity, and the dust attracted to their surfaces becomes a rich source of viruses and bacteria, so throw a cover over that TV and pretend it's broken!

I promise you'll discover extra scope to do all sorts of things for yourself you haven't had time to do before, such as massage, reading and taking long walks. Going without TV is much easier in the summer, when we focus on being outside, but even if you're doing the Plan in the depth of winter, surely you can last without the gogglebox for the Weekend.

> **! TOP TIP**
>
> If you can't possibly live without the TV now, or over the Weekend, at least try to avoid it after 8.30–9.00 p.m. This will give your nervous system a quiet hour to settle down before bed.

electric blanket

At least for the Weekend, dump your electric blanket – it creates a magnetic field that penetrates about 6 inches into the body. Go back to a hot-water bottle, if needed, during the three days – it's more natural. If you need an electric blanket after that, at least turn it off at the socket before you get into bed.

computers

PCs emit EMFs – in particular from the sides and the back of the VDU – so the advice from Powerwatch is to make sure you're sitting at arm's length from the screen. Laptops tend to be better, UNLESS you're working off the mains – then the transformer should be as far away from you as possible because of the high emissions. If you do use a laptop, work off battery power whenever possible (it's better for the equipment as well).

Whichever you have, for the sake of sleeping better in your build-up to the Plan, try to stop using the computer after 8 p.m. so you don't suffer from BBS – Busy Brain Syndrome. During the Weekend you certainly won't need to use a computer at all, so put it away!

hairdryers

High EMFs are emitted near the handle of a hairdryer and the higher the settings the higher the EMFs – even a few minutes can affect you. Don't wash your hair for the entire three days; then you won't need to dry it. Your body's natural excretions will be good for it, and you'll have covered it in oil from your self-massage anyway! Your hair will be in wonderful condition after that.

digital radio and alarm

Unplug your digital radio and/or alarm. You won't need to know the time constantly over the Weekend and waking up in silence is a real treat and quite enlightening if you're not used to it.

telephones

We all know about the debate around regular mobile-phone use, and whether it does or doesn't cause brain tumours. For the three days we're going to consider mobile phones a toxin. Even if they don't cause tumours, using a mobile for a long time always seems to drain me and make my ear hot!

Headaches, hot ears, fatigue and poor memory have also all been associated with using a *digital cordless* phone for extended periods. It's the base station that emits EMFs so, again, keep it as far away from you as possible when you're using the phone for a long chat.

Ordinary 'land lines' are absolutely fine, according to Powerwatch, but that isn't an excuse to chat away all weekend – remember, you're having 'quiet' time and don't need any outside chatter, stress or noise coming into your space. Cutting out that invasive ringing is one of the most empowering things you can do!

> **Put the phone on answerphone; tell people you're away; don't use it or go near it for the entire weekend. You no longer have a phone!**

microwaves

Microwaves don't emit EMFs, but Powerwatch is concerned about the lack of research on the effect of irradiating our food, as well as the health implications if an old microwave were to start leaking radiation. I got rid of mine a long time ago. (I gave it to my ex!)

There are two items on my 'avoid list' that aren't on the Powerwatch hit list, but I think it's worth doing without them, if only for the Weekend.

wristwatches

The batteries in wristwatches give off magnetic pulses several thousand times a second. We don't know the effect on our bodies, but take your watch off for three days – you won't need it all the time. Look at it only if, for example, you're timing a treatment.

underwired bras

The jury is out on these, but many people believe the metal acts as an antenna and re-radiates external EMFs, as well as microwave frequencies. You won't be using a microwave or a computer during the detox, but give your boobs a holiday as well and go without your underwired bra.

all those other toxins . . .

Unhealthy Relationships
Stressful Job
Stressful Home
Little or no Exercise
Little or no Fresh Air or
   Sunlight
Always-on-the-go

Don't Meditate
Don't do Breathing Exercises
Don't do Yoga or similar
No Time to just sit and be
No Time to relax
No Time for 'me'!

I would need another whole book to go into all of the above. Suffice it to say that you'll have placed a great big *'sorted' tick* by many of them by the end of the Weekend. The only three I can't help you with are the first three – only you can resolve these. But, after a weekend of opening your mind and having the time to 'just be', feelings about your job, relationships and home life will surface, and any answers needed will start popping into your head. The less time you spend experiencing the stress, the more you'll be able to address the cause. Just let the anxiety go and the solution will come all on its own. This is why people go on 'retreat' – shutting out all external influences so they can calmly re-evaluate their situation. They often come back with a whole new life plan in place! You'll be able to achieve the same clarity even without leaving home – provided all the 'noise' has been turned off and you get into techniques such as meditation.

All the other toxins on the list, from a lack of fresh air to finding time for 'me', will be addressed during the Plan. You'll be learning to meditate, breathe properly and follow an exercise routine that slows you right down – rather than winding you up. So, however many toxins you put an asterisk next to, don't worry: we can tackle the lot!

Your body is built to deal with toxins – it's constantly waging an internal battle against roving free radicals, bacteria and parasites. Toxicity only sets in when we take in more than we can get rid of, and the body's balance suffers. A strong immune system and efficient elimination routes will help us to cope with everyday exposure to toxins and stress, and that's why this 48-Hour Plan is so important. None of us can live a life of just breathing in pure air, just eating pure food and living entirely without electricity and other stimuli. But for three days we're going to get as close as we can to a natural life, in order to better arm our bodies for defence against living in the real world!

! TOP TIP

Did you know that listening to classical music first thing in the morning can increase your IQ by as much as 6 points? So put some classical music on instead of the over-stimulation of the TV or local pop station, fling open the windows (even in the winter), breathe deeply and then tell me you don't feel better, brighter and calmer.

You'll need more ideas to relax away those toxins, so in the next chapter we're going to have a look at baths – cold ones, hot ones, and in-between ones! As well as relaxing you and boosting your immune system, a good soak can also improve all sorts of conditions and complaints, as you'll soon discover. Read about the bath suggestions with an open mind, and pick one to try out as soon as possible.

8. H for Hydrotherapy

WARNING: If you suffer from fainting or dizzy spells, heart problems, or any other circulatory problem such as high or low blood pressure, read the chapter very carefully and avoid any of the suggestions if you have concerns. If in any doubt at all, always check with a medical expert.

what is hydrotherapy?

Hydrotherapy is described as the use of water in the treatment of disorders. It all started in the 1830s in Bavaria when a Roman Catholic priest called Sebastian Kneipp discovered that he, like so many others at the time, had tuberculosis. No remedies from orthodox medicine seemed to work, and after reading a book about 'water cures' he decided to give them a go. Despite having a raging fever, he jumped into an icy river and then jumped out again. He wrapped himself in warm blankets and went home to bed to sweat the poisons out. He had stimulated his immune system (remember the sluggish lymph?) into action; he repeated the treatment daily, and within weeks he had become stronger and was eventually cured. So the story goes. Today there is a Kneipp College and hydrotherapy is practised in many European hospitals and clinics.

It's a very useful therapy for the rehabilitation of arthritic or partially paralysed patients; but it's usually more widely seen as something a bit ridiculous that only the rich can afford at expensive health spas. But it should be taken seriously as an effective and beneficial technique.

I am not, for one moment, suggesting hydrotherapy as a TB cure or that you use it as a treatment for a medical condition. But I heartily recommend it as a *preventative* measure for strengthening the body's own natural healing powers. And, as has been discovered in health spas, the lymph and skin, and therefore cellulite, usually improve with hydrotherapy treatment.

benefits of hydrotherapy

Prevents colds and viruses.
Improves stamina.
Reduces stress levels.
Improves sleep.
Strengthens blood
    circulation.

Strengthens the nervous
    system.
Boosts the immune system.
Helps detoxify.
Boosts sluggish lymph.

In this section there are all sorts of different baths to choose from for your home spa. Have a good read through and see which one you fancy the sound of. If a temperature is given, this is only a guide – unless you happen to have a heat-proof thermometer about your person, just use your common sense and *listen to your body*. Nicely hot to some people could be dangerously scalding to others, so if in doubt start with the bath comfortably warm, and keep topping it up with hot water. Your *whole body* should be immersed, and you may want to have a book to hand, as you could be in there for a while! If you want to add any essential oils to a bath, use about three drops of each of your favourite essences.

types of baths

Warm Baths (90–95°F, 32.2–35°C) open the pores and create sweating, as well as helping to open the cells and release toxins. Warm baths can also help lower blood sugar, relieve painful joints and muscles, and improve colon peristalsis – moving your bowels! They are good for mild detoxing and mild colds and will be very beneficial to you over the Weekend. The hotter the water, the more profuse the sweating and the more dramatic the release of toxins. But, be careful, it could be too dramatic – over-stimulation can damage the body – so take it easy.

TIMING: Soak for 10–20 minutes.

> **WARNING: Please make sure you drink plenty of extra water before, during and after your bath as the heat and sweating will dehydrate your body.**

Cold Baths (55–65°F, 12.8–18.3°C) shock the system, stimulate it initially and then slow the heart right down. Cold baths are fantastic if you're very stressed, have 'Busy Brain Syndrome' or suffer from insomnia. They do the opposite of hot baths in that they can thin the blood, *increase* blood sugar and *reduce* colon peristalsis. In other words, cold baths slow your whole system right down as the blood rushes inwards to protect your organs.

TIMING: a quick dip of 6–30 seconds only!

WARNING: Do not have a cold bath if you suffer from heart problems, are feeling ill, run down or just coming down with something, however minor. Cold baths are for people in robust health!

baths with oils

You can add 3–10 drops of any one of these oils to a bath. Or use a combination of oils (to a total of 10 drops).

Lavender: Antibiotic, antiseptic, antidepressant, sedative, detoxifier, promotes healing. *If you buy only one essential oil, buy this one.*
Pine: Refreshing, relaxing and healing.
Camomile: Antispasmodic and calming.
Peppermint: Anti-inflammatory and antiseptic. Good for the digestion.
Melissa (lemon balm): Soothing and relaxing, sedative.
Thyme: Antiviral and antiseptic.
Lemon: Antiseptic, antibacterial and toning. Good for the lymphatic system.
Rosemary: Stimulates mentally and physically. Not really suitable for winding down.

medicated baths

Sea Salt Bath: Use this one to relax. The cooler the water and the shorter the time spent in the bath, the more it becomes a tonic. Add 3–5 lb (1.3–2.3 kg) of sea salt to a full bath.
Soak for 10–20 minutes.

Baking Soda Bath: For skin conditions such as eczema, hives or rashes. Baking soda (sodium bicarbonate) acts as a mild antiseptic, opens the pores and relieves itching and skin irritation. Add 1 lb (just under ½ kg) of baking soda to a full warm-to-cool bath.

Soak for 10–20 minutes.

Oatmeal Bath: For skin irritations, sunburn, chafing and windburn. Add 1–2 cups (125–250 g) of finely ground oatmeal to a full warm bath.

Soak for 15–30 minutes.

Apple Cider Vinegar Bath: Very good for detoxifying the body, helping the alkaline/acid balance and treating yeast infections such as thrush. Use organic or raw cider vinegar. Add 1–4 cups (250 ml–1 litre) to a full warm bath.

Soak for 15–20 minutes.

foot baths

Foot baths are very useful as relief for all sorts of symptoms that may come up during the Plan. Either sit on the edge of the bath, or get comfy on the sofa with your feet in a large plastic bowl.

hot foot bath

GOOD FOR:
Decongesting Internal Organs
Relieving Headaches
Warming the Body
Producing Sweating

Helping to Stop a Cold or Treat it
Relaxation
Tired Sore Feet (especially with mustard added!)
Chronically Cold Feet

A very simple but effective technique: fill your bath or a bowl with comfortably hot water to cover your feet and ankles. (Test it with a toe first to avoid scalding yourself.) Keep adding warm water to keep the temperature constant. Soak your feet for 10–20 minutes using any of the suggested oils. Finish by pouring cold water over the feet. Take it gently and make sure you're not sweating too much. Rest afterwards and drink plenty of water.

cold foot bath

GOOD FOR:

Tired Feet	Headache
Constipation	Nose Bleeds
Insomnia	Colds

This is absolutely brilliant if you're having trouble sleeping at night, especially if you're suffering from that Busy Brain Syndrome. Soak your feet in cold water until the cold becomes quite uncomfortable or till the feet start warming up. Whichever you can bear.

alternating hot/cold foot bath – lymph booster

GOOD FOR:

Circulation	Headache
Varicose Veins	High Blood Pressure
Insomnia	Immunity

Start by standing or soaking your feet for 1–2 minutes in hot water followed by 30 seconds in cold and keep alternating between the two for 15 minutes, ending on cold.

I tried this in an American health spa where they had added pebbles to the shallow pool so that the feet's reflexology points could be massaged as you walked from hot to cold, from cold to hot. The virus I was coming down with disappeared. If you live near a beach, you could add some small pebbles or stones to your bath for an added benefit! (But use a rubber mat underneath to prevent scratching the bath.)

TOP TIP FOR A QUICK 'FACE LIFT'

Cold water really tones and tightens the skin. Try using a hand-held shower on cool and blitz your face as close to the showerhead as possible. (BUT avoid the eyes if you've got the water on high.) Move the shower in a circular motion half a dozen times, first in a clockwise direction and then anti-clockwise. Finish by spraying your forehead for 30 seconds, then the temples, then the jawline. Pat skin dry with a fluffy warm towel.

TOP TIP: WIMP'S VERSION

Personally, I hate water pouring into my eyes so this is my wimpy version, and nearly as effective! Fill a basin with cold water. Either put your face into the cold water or soak a flannel in the basin and place it over the face. The water should be as cold as you can bear. Repeat half a dozen times and then pat skin dry.

Hydrotherapy can definitely strengthen your immune system. In the next chapter there'll be much more about the body's immunity and how to boost it.

9. I for **Immunity** and **Immune Response**

Bacteria and viruses are everywhere. We absorb them with our food and drink, and inhale them in the air we breathe. Our bodies are alive with them and, in fact, you're probably living with at least 1.2 kilos (over 2½ lb) of bacteria in your gut right now! Some of it essential to your well-being and some of it quite possibly damaging your health.

We only get sick if our immune system is weak; otherwise a human family would become extinct within months because there are so many germs around! The Naturopathic way of treatment, and the way I was trained, suggests that instead of killing the germs that might invade us, we should strengthen the blood and lymphatic systems so that the germs and viruses can't replicate and take over.

According to this philosophy, to kill germs without purifying the whole system is a bit like trying to keep a kitchen clean by bombarding every work surface with chemical germ-killers rather than flooding the room with fresh air and sunshine and washing all the cupboards out thoroughly. Interestingly, some scientists are now linking the enormous rise in asthma cases and allegies to us keeping our homes too artificially clean. We're also witnessing the rise in new 'superbugs' that seem impervious to the strongest antibiotics and disinfectants. Even with 21st-century living and our clean, carpeted homes, our immune systems seem to be getting weaker, not stronger.

We're now going to discover how we get ill, and discuss the impact of stress on the immune system. We'll also take a look at how the immune system may respond to a detox and how best to handle a 'healing crisis', should one arise. The rest of the book will show you how to keep your immune system healthy, through nutrition and lifestyle, so that hopefully it won't allow you to get ill in the first place! But first, how *do* you get ill?

how do I catch a cold or flu? a body's story

The virus or bacteria has to get into the body via one of the *entry routes* such as the nose and mouth. Imagine you're feeling very run down and overtired, and then someone sneezes near you in a confined space, for example on the Tube. You pick up the virus on one of your hands, touch your nose and, bingo, it enters through there into your throat. Once there, the virus pretends to be a protein so it can get into the throat cells. Healthy cells then becomes virus factories. Your system fights back as the *natural killer (NK) cells* that patrol the body spray the virus cells with poison.

Scavenger cells called *macrophages* now join the battle and, a bit like munching monsters, eat as many of the invaders and as much of the cell débris as they can. What they can't manage to consume is carried by the thousands of internal hair-like throat 'cilia' to be swallowed, coughed or sneezed out – which is what mucus is!

The body aches, the throat is sore and the lymph nodes swell up as the internal battle rages on. If the virus is a particularly nasty one, the macrophages will have to release *interleukins* – immune responders who will call for more reinforcements – which is when your body feels even worse, with aching limbs and joints. This is nature's way of telling you to slow down and rest so your body can concentrate on winning the war.

The interleukins turn the body's thermostat up to produce a fever. As the temperature rises the multiplying virus *slows down* and the immune cells start reproducing more quickly. The brain cells may swell as well, causing a headache. But this is *not* the time to take something to get rid of the headache because any analgesic will also lower the temperature – and to lower your temperature would be to give the virus a new lease of life. Viruses don't like heat.

The lymph (and now you'll see why getting the lymph moving is important) is carrying thousands of T and B cells. (*T cells* are produced and stored in the *thymus* gland. They attack a virus. *B cells* originate in the *bones* (up to 10 million of these cells are produced *an hour*!). They make antibodies.) One of these cells is waiting for the call to battle from dendritic – special communicating – cells. So, during the next stage of the illness, the dendritic cells gather fragments of the virus as prisoners of war and go in search of their secret weapon: the one T or B cell that will recognize the prisoner and clone it. A dendritic cell finally finds that one cell and docks. This particular T cell has been waiting an entire lifetime to fight this virus, and will now divide itself to become thousands more within hours. These T cells then launch into the bloodstream and the final battle commences – which you will recognize as swollen glands (lymph nodes), a bad cough, and so on.

Meanwhile, the B cell has also recognized the virus. B cells are not in the front line of the battle. Instead, they work in the arms factory producing millions of minute proteins that act as antibodies. They target the newborn viruses like heat-seeking missiles, lock on to and paralyse them. The virus is wiped out.

New cells will grow back replacing the damaged ones, and most of the T cells will die having done the job they were born to do. A few will survive as 'memory' cells so that if the same virus reappears it will be zapped immediately. Unfortunately, viruses mutate and come back in new disguises!

Isn't the body amazing? Hopefully, this story has helped explain *why* keeping T, B and NK cells healthy and abundant is so important. The rest of the book will explain *how*.

psycho neuro immunology

Psycho Neuro Immunology (PNI) basically means 'a bridge between psychology and the nervous and immune systems'. We need to understand a little about this new science if we're going to give ourselves a resilient immune system.

Very recently scientists found a nerve cell 'communicating' with an immune cell – a lymphocyte – in a petri dish in a lab experiment. For the first time scientists accepted what complementary therapists have believed for years. There *is* a link between the brain – and emotions – and the immune system. This, they deduced, would affect the way lymphocytes behave, and PNI was born.

In a healthy person there are six sites full of lymphocytes, NK cells and all the other cells specifically waiting to fight disease. They're found where the lymphocyte production plants are located: in the liver, spleen, lymph nodes, large intestine, small intestine and tonsils.

what decreases nk cell activity

Chronic Stress   Lack of Exercise
Chronic Anger   Exhaustion
Over Exercise   Poor Nutrition

But one of the biggest enemies for NK cells is *stress*. Constant physical or mental stress eventually weakens them and reduces their numbers. Along comes a virus and, if there aren't enough of the warrior cells around to tackle the invader, we get sick.

the four types of stress

Poisonous People: Friends, boss, partner, clients, etc. People who constantly make you feel angry or worthless. Give them up!

Doing Too Much: The hamster-on-the-treadmill scenario. Pace yourself.

Sleep Deprivation: Difficult if you're a mother of young children. (Some self-help techniques coming up.)

Life-changing Events Too Close Together: Don't make big decisions for a year after a crisis, e.g.: don't decide to change your job just after a bereavement.

Strangely enough though, *short* bursts of the right kind of stress *increase* the activity of the natural killer cells. It's been discovered that fairground rides, thrills and spills, even the stress of falling in love, can all increase the amount of NK cells in the body. This could be the excuse you've been waiting for to tap the child inside you, join your kids on the roller coaster and benefit your health at the same time.

In one study, cancer patients on chemotherapy were given relaxation and visualization exercises to help them cope with the side effects of their treatment. Five years later doctors discovered that the patients who routinely practised relaxation techniques and had regular 'treats' such as massage had a higher count of NK cells, a stronger immune system, and a longer survival rate than those who didn't. Professor Stafford Lightman, Director of the Research Centre for Neuroendocrinology, Bristol Royal Infirmary, says, 'There is no evidence that the mind can cure disease, but the evidence suggests that the mind can alter the progression of the disease or your *susceptibility* to disease.'

The body's equivalent of an opiate – a feel-good drug that makes you happy and kills pain – is an endorphin. (Endorphins are believed by some to be up to *200 times more powerful than morphine*!) They are natural chemicals that tell the NK cells where to 'hang out' to fight infection. To increase your endorphin production, and therefore your NK cell count, you need to exercise and do things that make you very happy and relaxed – regularly!

There are other ways of increasing NK cell activity, which we will be looking at during the Weekend Plan. Tick the ones on the list below that you already include in your life and put an asterisk next to the ones you might like to try out during the Plan.

Exercise (a minimum of five 20–30 minute sessions a week)
Massage
Love
A Pet
Joy/Happiness
Support
Sex
Doing Things You Enjoy
Crying
Short Spells of Acute Stress (fairground ride, bungee jump, etc.)
Relaxing
Meditation
Yoga
Good Nutrition

immune response and a healing crisis

Finally, since we're looking at the body's immune system, we need to consider how it responds to sudden changes. Releasing too much toxicity too quickly can make you feel terrible and, if you're already unwell, make you sicker. So look out for any symptoms during your detox that may appear as a 'healing crisis'.

The best thing to do if you suffer from an immune response is to rest and increase your food and water intake. Headaches and feeling tired during a detox are the most common symptoms, but they don't last long and have usually gone completely by the third day. Some patients on a detox experience cold-like symptoms or sinus congestion but, again, these usually clear up within two to three days. Others suffer from bloating or constipation. All these symptoms are a sign that your body is trying to adjust to its new diet. It *will* adjust, given a little time and some encouragement, as long as you don't rush things.

Don't forget that to cleanse itself your body needs to use every exit route it has. So welcome that cold as a useful detoxifier and treat that heavy period as a sign that the body is unloading toxins like mad. (There is more information on exit routes and how to use them in chapter 15.)

what to take during a healing crisis

Constipation: Apple, honey, liquorice, strawberries or dried fruit such as prunes or apricots.

Bloating: Hot water with a slice of lemon, dill or fennel tea.

Wind: Camomile, dill, fennel or peppermint tea, or warm vinegar with a little honey.

Nausea or Vomiting: Fennel or peppermint tea, and barley water. Once the symptoms have gone, drink warm water with lemon juice to rebalance everything.

Diarrhoea: Barley water, peppermint tea.

Headache: A dab of lavender essential oil on the temples. A mustard footbath is also a traditional remedy.

Colds and Flu: Vitamin C + zinc supplement. LARGE DOSES OF VITAMIN C CAN CAUSE A VERY LOOSE TUMMY, SO REDUCE THE DOSAGE OR STAY NEAR A LOO. IF YOU'RE ON ANY MEDICATION OR HAVE A HISTORY OF KIDNEY COMPLAINTS CONSULT YOUR DOCTOR BEFORE TAKING VITAMIN C SUPPLEMENTS.

Sore Throat: Zinc in lozenge form.

Cough: Fresh honey and lemon mixed in a little water.

Spots: Dab on tea tree essential oil. Drink more water.

Cold Sores: A few drops of undiluted lemon juice two or three times a day. Melissa (lemon balm oil) essential oil works for me – it's fantastic for nipping them in the bud.

Insomnia: Camomile tea, a few drops of lavender oil on the pillow (don't let it get near your eyes), valerian tincture drops (diluted in water), or a *cold* water footbath.

Heavy Period: Warm water with lemon juice, peppermint or camomile tea.

And these spices are also very useful for various complaints:

Chilli: Good for sweating, helps detox the body and aids decongestion. Fresh chilli is rich in vitamin C.

Cayenne: Invigorates and warms the circulation, improves the digestion and acts as a lung decongestant.

Cinnamon: Good for nausea and indigestion, and helps with diarrhoea.

Turmeric: Improves the digestive function; helps with inflammation and diarrhoea.

Garlic: Useful against colds, infections and intestinal parasites. Helps keep the blood thin and lowers blood pressure. It's one of nature's natural antibiotics.

Ginger: Supports the digestion, relieves nausea (try ginger tea) and stimulates the circulation. Good for painful digestion, colic and diarrhoea. It's warming, anti-viral and essential for a successful detox.

So now you know how your immune system works and how to keep it healthy and strong. We all have a pretty good idea that optimum nutrition and a lack of stress is vital in keeping us fit and well but exercise also plays a role in ensuring those NK cells are armed and ready for battle. The next chapter is devoted to exercise – there are some simple suggestions that you can easily work into your Weekend Plan, even if you've never exercised before. But, more importantly, you'll discover how exercise can benefit not just your immune system, but your whole body, mind and spirit as well.

10.
E for Exercise

There is no doubt that regular exercise promotes weight loss. In fact, the best nutrition in the world won't help the body's ability to burn fat efficiently unless it goes hand in hand with exercise. The two need each other for the best results, and I speak from personal experience!

> If you were to walk briskly for 45 minutes a day, four times a week, you would lose 18 lbs (over 8 kg) in a year without changing your diet!

We know that leading a sedentary lifestyle and carrying too much weight can lead to a myriad of health problems, from chronic backache and joint problems to heart disease, but the other important reason to take up exercise, especially during the Plan, is to improve your *emotional* health: *de-stressing* as well as detoxing. As we have seen, too much stress becomes *distress* and has a negative effect on the body unless we can find an outlet for it – and exercise is one of the very best.

While meditation techniques and yoga exercises help still the mind, what the body also needs to combat stress is some 'fight or flight' activity: 20–40 minutes of aerobic exercise causes the release of endorphins, those 'happy hormones' we should all treat ourselves to. Endorphins have been found to stay in the blood for as long as two hours after exercise, accounting for the well-known 'high' regular exercisers talk about. Aerobic exercise – such as brisk walking or cycling – is considered the best for endorphin release because it's an extended endurance activity requiring an increased use of oxygen. (*Anaerobic* exercise – such as sprinting – is higher in intensity, but shorter in duration, and means the muscles are working with *less* than the usual supply of oxygen. That's not what I'm recommending here.)

You don't have to train for a marathon to get the required effect – almost any exercise will do as long as it's fairly repetitive and continuous and lasts for at least 20 minutes, but preferably nearer 40 minutes. You should be sweating lightly. How long it takes for the endorphins to kick in depends on the type of exercise and the individual. Some experience endorphin highs by swimming in the local pool for half an hour, while others find that just playing loud music at home and dancing their socks off for 20 minutes will do the trick. Brisk walking with a dog for 40 minutes has a remarkable effect on stress levels, while activities like kick-boxing do wonders for getting rid of any pent-up anger. Regular aerobic exercise, as well as practices like yoga, has been found to reduce the heart rate and blood pressure dramatically in only three months. Stress symptoms like anxiety, depression and anger can disappear within 20 minutes of starting an exercise session – from day one! Most regular exercisers also report having more energy generally, sleeping better and experiencing a clearer mind. Weight loss and better self-esteem are usually thrown in for good measure.

I appreciate how impossible it is for working mums to fit any more into their overcrowded day but, for the Weekend at least, do try some of the suggestions. You may well find that once you've started and felt the benefits you *will* find the time to continue post-Plan, even if it's only power-walking to the shops with the pushchair!

You don't need to dig out that trendy gym gear that has been lurking in a drawer for ages, unless you really want to! You don't need to join an expensive health club and start pounding on a treadmill surrounded by people wearing designer tracksuits. It's a lot simpler than that, as you'll see once you've taken off your watch and stopped saying to yourself, 'But I haven't got time!'

reasons to exercise

Increases immunity.

Reduces stress.

Produces endorphins.

Reduces weight.

Prevents heart disease.

Lowers cholesterol levels.

Prevents osteoporosis.

Prevents back problems.

Strengthens bones and
joints.

Prevents hypertension.

Prevents diabetes.

WARNING: If you have never exercised regularly before, or have not been active for some time, have a health condition or are seriously overweight, please build up very slowly to 30 minutes a day, even if you start at only 5 minutes a day. And please always check with your doctor if you have any doubts.

suggested aerobic exercises

Walking   Gym Work
Power-Walking   Kick-Boxing
Dancing   Tennis
Cycling   Jogging
Swimming   Rebounding
Local Sports Centre Activities
  such as Step Classes

For the Weekend Plan, I am recommending only brisk walking as an aerobic exercise, because it is safe for all. If you regularly jog or go to the gym, then please carry on with whatever you usually do, provided you have the energy for it. If you have a bike and feel like cycling, go ahead. You choose, it's your time.

The important thing is to do whatever *you enjoy*, as long as you get moving. Or try something that reaches the child in you, such as rollerblading or whizzing along on a microscooter, or flying a kite. Anything that gets you moving for a minimum of 30 minutes a day over the three days.

walking

Walking is just the best exercise! It strengthens the heart and lungs and works all the lower-body muscles. It's a weight-bearing activity, so it'll improve bone density, but it's also low impact, so puts less stress on the joints than running or jogging. Walking is the most frequently prescribed form of exercise when it comes to preventing conditions such as osteoarthritis and osteoporosis, as well as chronic backache – which plagues 10 million people a year in the UK alone.

According to the experts, just *being* a woman causes problems for the human skeleton. Pregnancy, lifting young children, carrying heavy shopping, housework and gardening all put a tremendous strain on bones and joints. And those of us who spend anything from 25 to 40 hours a week working at a computer and then slump in front of the TV when we get home, because we're so exhausted, are heading for trouble – and so are our children.

'Our children lead such sedentary lifestyles that in later life they are at high risk of back pain, heart disease, osteoporosis and obesity,' warns Colin Jones, the Chief Executive of Back-Care, the charity for healthier backs. 'If muscles, bones and tendons fall into disuse they will start to grumble and groan, so we need to keep them moving.' Dr Mike Hurley, Reader in Physiotherapy at King's College, London, agrees. 'It's a myth that people will wear down their joints by walking on them – people are doing themselves the greatest damage by sitting in a chair and doing nothing.'

So get walking! The faster you walk the more energy you use, till eventually it's easier to start running (for which you *would* need special shoes). *Walking* at this high speed will actually burn more calories than *running* at the same speed, and will really work your lungs, heart and muscles. Remember, the more you sweat, the more toxins are coming out. But make sure the speed you're walking at still allows you to talk comfortably – that's an indication that you're exercising *aerobically*. You should be walking very purposefully, as if you had a bus to catch, as opposed to just dawdling along.

If you're spending the Weekend in the country, you'll have an endless choice of walks over hills, through woodland areas or along coastal routes if by the sea. Make sure you're dressed in sensible walking shoes and waterproof clothes, and take all the usual safety precautions: take along plenty to drink, food, a compass, a map, etc.

If you're in a city, find a big park, or a river, or a hilly area – even if it's just a steep road – and go for it! Walking uphill will work your heart more, make you breathe harder, sweat more and burn more calories. And, believe it or not, walking *downhill* also increases aerobic activity because you're using different muscles as shock absorbers. So try and find a hilly area if you want the hardest work-out.

! TOP TIPS FOR WALKING DURING THE
● WEEKEND PLAN

Make sure you've first warmed up your muscles by doing
some stretching (or yoga) exercises.
Keep your head and shoulders relaxed.
Wear loose comfortable clothes and good trainers or shoes.
Take a waterproof instead of an umbrella, to free yourself up.
Swing your arms to get your heart pumping even more.
Towards the end of your walk, slow down and cool down.
Stretch all the muscles you've been using and take your
time, don't rush.

yoga

Yoga is an excellent de-stresser and detoxer. No matter how
unfit, how old, how overweight, or how anti-exercise you are,
you can practise yoga. Don't be put off by the super-fit celeb-
rities who can twist their bodies into apparently impossible
positions. A 5,000-year-old science, yoga was designed to unite
body, mind and spirit. It combines movement, relaxation,
breathing and meditation. Regular practice will strengthen the
body, increase your flexibility and develop a sense of calm,
mental focus and well-being.

long-term benefits of yoga

Improves oxygen supply to the blood.
Benefits circulation.
Less risk of joint problems than other forms of exercise.
Relieves asthma and hyperventilating.
Stimulates digestive system and reduces constipation.

Helps blood pressure, headaches and back pain.
Tones muscles, so helps with cellulite and saggy skin!
Helps with sleep problems and stress.

If you're used to doing yoga regularly, you can start each day of the Plan with six rounds of Sun Salutations instead of, or as well as, the exercises listed below. But if you've never tried yoga before and have always fancied it, have a go at some, or all, of these suggestions over the Weekend and hopefully you'll want to continue with a qualified teacher. There are also some excellent videos and books available if you want to learn more about yoga. (You don't need fancy gear to give it a try — just wear comfortable clothes and take your shoes off!)

These yoga exercises have been compiled by my yoga teacher, Patricia Haygarth — the slimmest, fittest granny you've ever seen! Patricia is a shining example of why we should all be practising yoga. She's incredibly supple, looks healthy and vibrant and doesn't have an ounce of loose skin or fat on her body.

Start off with these simple postures (or *asanas*, as they are called) and just enjoy them. There are only a handful of them, plus warm-up and relaxation. It may help to practise with a friend so you can encourage each other! But doing it on your own is still very rewarding. If you're completely new to yoga, allow yourself plenty of time to get your head around these suggested *asanas*. (The Sanskrit names of the postures are given in brackets.) Bear in mind:

the points to remember

Yoga movements are based on elongating the spine, so whichever posture you're in, *think tall* and stretch your spine — this usually means lifting the chest and breathing as deeply as you can.

Once you're in a posture, *relax* into the stretch – paying attention especially to the shoulders and nape of the neck.

Never strain your back – respect your body and listen to what it's telling you.

Avoid fast or jerky movements – try to flow gently from one position to the next.

Don't forget to breathe when you're in a posture, starting with about four breaths and gradually increasing this number as you become more confident.

The quality of breathing during practice is very important. Watch out for this. If you're struggling or forcing your body your breathing will become laboured. When you're calm, centred and sensitive to your body, it'll get into the position easier, and this is what we're aiming for in yoga.

If you stretch one side of the body, always repeat on the other side to keep your practice even. Hold for the same length of time on each side.

Finish your session with a minimum of 10 minutes' relaxation in the 'Corpse pose'.

1. WARM-UP

Use an old towel or a yoga mat to sit and lie on. Begin by lying down with feet apart; your toes should be rolling away from your heels, and your arms a little away from your body with the palms of your hands facing the ceiling. Close your eyes. Just allow the body to become quiet and still for about 2–3 minutes, releasing any tension you find, particularly in the hips, shoulders, chin and jawline. Have a really good, long stretch with your arms over your head.

Then come up to a comfortable sitting position on the floor, cross-legged, with your spine straight and your shoulders relaxed. Gently drop your head to your chest, stretching your neck. Take a few breaths and then gently turn your head twice to the right and twice to the left to ease any stiffness there. Don't take your neck back. Just roll your head from side to side a few times. Then interlock your fingers and stretch your arms out ahead of you, palms outwards. Take them up and over your head reaching as high as you can. Stretch the whole upper body to the left and then to the right, and release your arms. Then interlock your fingers behind your back and stretch your body forward as far as you can, keeping your head in line with your spine. Hold then release.

Then move on to some *leg lifts, which strengthen abdominal, back and leg muscles*. Lie on your back on the floor, arms by your sides and neck long (point the chin down towards your chest). Keep toes flexed towards your face. As you inhale extend the right heel and lift the right leg as high as you can. Keep the leg straight. Hold for a few breaths and then release on an exhalation. Repeat with the left leg. Alternate as many times as is comfortable. As one leg lifts the other one is also working by keeping itself strong along the floor with toes also flexed.

2. FORWARD BEND (*PASCHIMOTHANASANA*)

This is a seated posture, which is a complete stretch for the back of the body, massages all the abdominal organs and relieves constipation. It also counteracts obesity and strengthens and stretches the hamstrings (backs of thighs).

Sit with your legs straight out in front of you, with your toes flexed towards your face. Stretch your trunk upward, keeping the spine elongated, and raise your arms above the head as you inhale deeply. As you exhale, bend forward from the hips. Reach forward towards your feet and bring your chest down towards your thighs – only go as far as you feel comfortable. You are aiming towards your toes – take hold of your thighs, shins, or ankles – whatever you can reach. Hold as long as is comfortable, and then inhale and stretch your arms and body back up. Repeat several times for maximum benefit. Then lie down and rest your back.

3. LOCUST (*SALABHASANA*)

This is one of the back bends, which increase flexibility, rejuvenate the spinal nerves, and bring a rich blood supply to the vertebrae. This particular one also strengthens the lower back, abdomen, thighs, and hips, and stimulates the adrenal glands and kidneys.

Lie on your tummy with your legs together and your toes pointing away from the body. Place your arms at the sides of your body, with the palms down. As you inhale lift both legs up and pull your arms back and away from the body, raising your chest and arms off the floor. Hold for several breaths, then release. Repeat once or twice more. Then rest.

Follow this with two inverted postures – the most beneficial of all asanas, because the heart is higher than the head, increasing the supply of oxygen to the brain and allowing the heart to rest, as gravity helps to return de-oxygenated blood to it.

4. DOG HEAD DOWN (*ADHO MUKHA SVANASANA*)

This stretches the back, legs and ankles, and massages the abdominal muscles.

In a kneeling position place your hands on the floor so that they're immediately below the shoulders, just in front of you. On an exhalation, raise your hips into the air, lifting your knees off the floor, to form an inverted 'V'. Press your chest towards the floor, while lifting and pointing your tailbone upwards. Drop your head towards the floor. Lift as high as you can, and then release your heels towards the floor, giving a good stretch to the legs. Don't force your heels down – they may not touch the floor for many years! Keep your arms and legs as straight as you can. Hold for as long as is comfortable, and then release. Repeat.

5. HALF SHOULDERSTAND (*ARDHA SARVANGASANA*)

> **WARNING: This is potentially a very beneficial exercise, but do not attempt it if you've ever had any neck problems.**

This one benefits the whole body. The thyroid gland is massaged together with the other endocrine glands: so it's fantastic for the immune and nervous systems, and brings peace and stillness to the mind.

Lie on your back. Using your arms for support, raise your legs and buttocks into the air, while keeping your legs together. Place your hands on your buttocks to support your back. Your arms will be at an angle from the body. Press your neck to the floor AND DO NOT, WHATEVER YOU DO, TURN YOUR HEAD TO THE RIGHT OR LEFT. This can be really dangerous. Try to hold the position for several minutes and when ready, roll each vertebra back to the floor, from the top of the spine to the bottom, keeping your head on the floor if possible. Extend your legs and rest for several minutes.

(Some yoga teachers say that if everyone did this exercise every day for 10–20 minutes, no one would ever need to diet!)

This should be followed by the Bridge as a counterpose to stretch your back out.

6. THE BRIDGE (*SETU BANDHASANA*)

This stretches and strengthens the neck and loosens the shoulders, and improves spinal flexibility.

Lie on your back with your knees bent, your heels close to your buttocks and your feet as far apart as your hips. With your arms at your sides, inhale and raise your hips, rolling each vertebra up until you're resting on your shoulders. Bring your hands on to the back with the fingers pointing towards the spine and the thumbs around the waist. Your feet, shoulders, neck, back of the head and upper arms are supporting your body. Feel the stretch in your thighs, back, neck and shoulders. Keep your knees, legs and feet in line. Breathe deeply and hold as long as is comfortable. Release by slowly rolling down.

7. FINAL RELAXATION – THE CORPSE (*SAVASANA*)

Just as it's important to begin every asana session with a period of relaxation, it's also essential to finish with one of about 10 minutes. This gives the physical and mental energy released by the asanas an opportunity to circulate properly.

Lie flat on your back with your feet apart, and your toes rolling away from the heels. Have your arms at your sides and slightly away from your body, with the palms facing up. Make sure your head is straight and your neck is long. Allow your mind to help the body relax and repeat mentally to yourself as you travel through the body, beginning with your toes, 'I relax my toes . . . my toes are relaxed. I relax my feet and ankles . . . my feet and ankles are relaxed. I relax my legs . . .' and so on, until you reach your head and finally your mind. Relax. Relax. Relax. Stay there as long as you like, you might even fall asleep!

Allow your breathing to deepen and bring yourself back,

stretching your legs and arms and then rolling to the right –
stay there in a foetus position for a couple of minutes before
coming up to a comfortable cross-legged position. With your
hands on your knees, keep your eyes closed and just spend a
minute or two following your breathing, breathing *in* peace
and breathing *out* love. Need I say more?

11. R for Rhythms

Because nature's rhythms affect each and every one of us in different ways, this chapter is one of the most useful ones if you want to get the very best out of your three-day break – and one, I hope, that you'll come back to over the Weekend.

Whether it's the 24-hour cycle of day and night or the cycle of changing seasons, the natural rhythms of the planet we live on have a profound impact on each and every one of us. We've seen how considering the seasons and the moon cycles is important in planning when to have your weekend away. Here I want to concentrate on thinking about organizing your activities on those detoxing days. Every cell in your body is ruled by light and, according to Chinese medicine, each organ in the body functions much better at certain *times* of the day or night. So imagine how much we could benefit healthwise if we were to follow our natural rhythms a little more than we usually do and work *with* them rather than against them!

Of course, being as close to nature as possible would entail going to sleep when it gets dark and waking up when it gets light. Wouldn't it be wonderful to go with the flow and sleep for 14 hours a night in the winter and manage on far less in the summer when there is so much more to get up for? It's not easy to do in the 21st century, when even the birds are confused by artificial light and continue to sing through the night in built-up areas! But it's very possible to do during your three-day Plan.

Any mother reading this is probably thinking that I'm barking mad. How on earth can a parent get even eight uninterrupted hours of sleep a night? That's why it's so important for you to have a child-free weekend. Just for once in your life you *will* be able to get the amount of sleep your body needs. You *will* be able to try eating at different times of the day to see what it feels like and you *will* be able to go with the flow.

If you can't change your routine by going to bed and getting up any earlier *after* the 48-Hour Plan don't worry – just try it for one weekend. Be utterly selfish and do what you want to do, when you want to do it. The background information and suggested timetable below is just that – information and suggestions!

body clocks

We have various internal clocks that regulate different bodily functions throughout the day. The most important is the 'circadian rhythm' (from the Latin 'circa' – about – and 'dies' – day) – it's a 24-hour cycle that influences the important biological processes such as body temperature, hormone production and waking and sleeping. Problems with the circadian clock can cause all sorts of disorders – one of the most obvious is jet lag.

According to our circadian rhythm, there are two natural periods of sleep: between 10 p.m. and midnight, and between 1.30 and 2 p.m. So on all those occasions when you've blamed your lunch for that early afternoon slump, this drowsiness may well have been more due to your circadian rhythm, rather than to what you've eaten – although that plays a part as well! The

Spanish obviously know something we don't, and I for one would heartily recommend a short siesta after lunch if that's what your body tells you it needs – especially during the 48-Hour Plan.

! TOP TIP FOR MOTHERS, SHIFT WORKERS AND
• ALL-NIGHT PARTIERS

If you *have* been up all night, 15-minute naps throughout the day are much more suited to our natural circadian rhythm than a longer sleep – so try to grab a quick quarter of an hour when you can, rather than sleeping for longer and throwing your body clock out of synch even more.

The hormone cortisol, produced by the adrenal glands for fight or flight, also rises and falls according to a 24-hour clock. Cortisol levels in the blood peak at the start of the day at around 7 a.m. but dip in the late afternoon or early evening when nature intended our hunting activities to slow down. They remain low during the night when we slept around fires which scared off wild beasts.

Body temperature follows a completely different 24-hour pattern. It increases through the day and reaches a *high* point in the late afternoon or early evening (a great time for sex and exercise!) and then decreases to a *low* a few hours after midnight: between two and four in the morning. There are more natural deaths, suicides and episodes of depression during those hours than at any other time of the day or night. I can't help thinking there must be a connection.

There are good times to carry out certain activities for your body processes. If we eat, sleep and eliminate at the optimum time, even if it is only for three days, we'll reap the benefits of nature's vitality and strength.

Here is an example of a 24-hour clock incorporating Indian Ayurvedic principles, the Chinese method of linking certain organs to certain times of the day, our natural circadian rhythm and the way the human body has evolved over the last few thousand years. I'm not suggesting that this clock should be a blueprint to be followed religiously during the Weekend, because I believe that you should only do what you want with 'your' time without having to refer to a rigid timetable. But I hope you'll find it useful and interesting, and at least try some of the suggested time slots (also before or after your 48-hour break). It's your plan and your choice!

suzi's optimum body clock

morning

6–7 a.m.: According to all the research I've done, one of the keys to a healthier life is waking up at the right time and in the right way. Ideally, this should be without an alarm clock and around sunrise, which could be as early as 4 a.m. in the summer, or as late as 8 a.m. in the winter. Some of us 'owls' find it very difficult to become 'larks', but these tips have helped me change from a lifetime of staying up late to someone who can't bear to miss a second of sunlight!

You may, initially, need an alarm clock to wake up at such an ungodly hour while your system adjusts to the new schedule. Set it for 7 a.m. at the very latest if you want to become a lark. Always get out of bed no matter how you feel, put some classical or new-age music on, and get on with your daily routine. By the evening you should feel tired enough to go to bed earlier than normal, enabling you to reset your biological clock. At first you *will* feel tired and slightly jet-lagged but eventually – I promise – you'll feel better when you wake up and realize that you suddenly have all this extra 'me' time in the day!

! TOP TIP FOR RELUCTANT LARKS

If your hours are really out of synch with nature's rhythms, and a sudden change would be too difficult to cope with, instead try adjusting by setting your alarm clock progressively earlier. Every three or four days move your waking time ahead by 10 or 15 minutes. Gradually you will start feeling sleepy earlier in the evening and your body will soon adjust to its new rhythm.

This is the time of the day to have soothing music on in the background, to do stretching and breathing exercises and have some quiet time, even if you have to hide in the bathroom to accomplish this!

Having a drink of warm water and lemon now, instead of tea or coffee, will really wake up the digestive system and, because **5–7 a.m. is large intestine time**, this is the perfect time to move your bowels. Having a poo as soon as you can after waking allows your body to get rid of toxins and waste that have been accumulating in your system overnight. Starting a new day with clean insides is not something many of us can find the time to do.

But if you lock yourself in the bathroom and just sit there for 5 to 10 minutes every morning, the bowel will eventually do the job it's supposed to do and get into a regular and natural cycle.

7.30–8.30 a.m.: This is the time of day when exercise will best boost your energy levels. Try a 20-minute gentle jog, or 30 minutes of brisk walking, outside in the fresh air and sunlight. This will really wake you up and speed up your metabolism which, in turn, will promote weight loss. If it's winter you may well want to move this session to a little later when it's lighter, and wrap up warmly! If the weather is really foul, you could stay inside and do the suggested yoga exercises.

8–9 a.m.: A good time to moisturize and massage your skin. Following a skin-brushing session, have a warm bath or shower and then do the suggested self-massage technique.

Between 7 and 9 a.m. is stomach time, so start the day with a hearty breakfast. You are 'breaking a fast', so the body needs lots of nutrients at this time, in the form of fruit, grains and nuts. Warm porridge will sustain you for longer during the winter months and the smoothie (recipe in chapter 14) will keep you going during spring, summer and even autumn.

Try and eat breakfast within an hour of exercise. This means the carbohydrate content is converted to glucose quickly, rather than stored as fat, and will go straight to the muscles that need it.

10 a.m.–midday: The best time for doing research or admin – obviously not during the Plan! But a great time for reading, relaxing and thinking!

Midday: The body needs a snack because your brain

has used nearly a quarter of the available glucose by now. Seeds and nuts with dried fruit will be the best snacks for maximum brain energy. (This is also the most beneficial time to have a cup of coffee if you are still having just the one a day!)

Go for a walk around this time as your body temperature and energy levels will be starting to decline between now and 2 p.m.

afternoon

1–3 p.m. is small intestine time, so now is the best time for the absorption of nutrients. Make sure your lunch is packed full of vitamins and minerals from fresh fruit and vegetables, seeds and nuts, pulses and brown rice.

2 p.m.: The usual time for our natural body rhythm to slow right down. Have a catnap of no more than 15 minutes, if you can.

Between 3 and 5 p.m. is bladder time, and between 5 and 7 p.m. is kidney time, so drink extra water between 3 and 7 p.m. to help flush your system. (But remember to have the right amount and to leave a gap before eating your evening meal.) This is also the worst time of the day for sugar cravings. A glass of fruit juice, or a cup of herbal tea, and a snack of seeds, nuts and fruit will help stabilize your blood-sugar levels.

6 p.m.: The best time to go to the gym as your body temperature has risen to its highest level and your muscles will be nice and warm. During the 48-Hour Plan, this is a good time to go for a 30-minute brisk walk or do the yoga exercises, as you may want to avoid the gym.

The best time to eat supper is between 6 and 8 p.m. so that your body has a fighting chance of breaking the food down and assimilating its nutrients before you go to sleep (when it should be repairing your cells rather than digesting food). Nature is expecting us to ease off from our 'hunting' activities at this time of the day so we should eat ideally not much later than 6 p.m. so that digestion would be completed by around 10 p.m. Late meals require an increase in metabolism when we should be slowing down, and this can disrupt your sleep pattern.

You'll be pleased to hear that alcohol has *less* of a negative effect now than at any other time of the day because the blood absorbs it more slowly in the evening as there is more food in the system. So if you're going to have a drink (NOT during the Weekend), now's the time.

7–9 p.m. is Circulation Sex time (in Chinese medicine) – the best time for the reproductive organs. Interestingly, in Western medicine this time slot has also been found to be the best time for sex because sperm production peaks at around 4 p.m. and ovulation normally takes place between 3 and 7 p.m. on an ovulating day! It's a good time for sex even if you are *not* trying for a baby as the body will be winding down and de-stressing.

9–10 p.m. is a good time to cleanse – so a bath, steam or massage would really benefit you around now. It's also important to unwind, so make it a relaxing bath, meditate or do some yoga exercises. Do anything that helps slow you right down such as reading, talking, listening to soothing music or even having a gentle walk around the block.

Watching TV at this time is not brilliant because it excites the nervous system, even if the programme is low-key. This also applies to working or sorting out your bills. You don't want to be doing anything at this time that gets your brain going. **Try to avoid watching TV or doing any work after 8.30–9 p.m.** This will allow the system a quiet hour to settle down before bed! (And of course you won't be doing either during the Weekend, will you?)

10–11 p.m.: If you want to bound out of bed early in the morning, you're going to need to be in bed by around 10 p.m. the night before. If you've had a relaxing, stimulus-free evening, this will be much easier. Don't get agitated if you can't sleep, just relax.

From 11 p.m.–3 a.m. is gall bladder and liver time, so the body's best chance of cleansing and repairing itself is going to be during those hours. If you know the expression 'an hour's sleep before midnight is worth two hours *after* midnight', these organ times make sense. If you want strong collagen and, therefore, good skin it's important to get as much deep sleep as possible before 3 a.m. As you know from experience, the later you get to bed the lighter and more restless your sleep is. Too many nights like that and eventually chronic fatigue sets in, with mood swings and a dull complexion.

Research has also shown that people who are regularly denied sufficient sleep have a reduced number of natural killer cells in their blood to fight infections. It's thought that sleep is needed for the brain to 'talk' to these immune cells, which may have become weakened during the day.

what sleep does for you

Boosts the immune system.
Rests the heart and central nervous system.
Enables all the organs to repair themselves.
Repairs muscles.
Nocturnal growth hormones repair the skin.
Improves mood.
Makes us brighter!

Your bedroom should be a sleeping room, so avoid watching TV or working in it. You should start feeling sleepy, naturally, when darkness falls. If you don't, a pre-bedtime cup of soothing camomile tea or snacks such as bananas, cottage cheese, or turkey – anything full of the amino acid tryptophan – will help you sleep better and shouldn't interfere with your digestion too much. (None of these are on the menu during the 48-hour detox, so use one of the bath suggestions in chapter 8 instead.)

If you can't get to sleep, instead of putting the light on and reading, which will stimulate the brain, rest with your eyes closed and adopt a 'I don't care if I don't sleep' attitude. Recognize that falling asleep is out of your control and is up to nature – *trying* to sleep doesn't work, and nor does counting sheep!

It's important to arrange to do nothing during the three day Plan so that it won't matter if you don't get to sleep till the middle of the night – you've got all the following day to catch up! Even if you are *not* sleeping, your body is still getting much-needed rest and it's far better to be in bed with the lights out during this early and important part of the night than to be up and about. Remember, this Weekend is all about getting back in touch with nature, having a completely stress-free three days, and looking after yourself.

And, as you're now well aware, the organ we need to nurture as much as possible during any detox plan is the liver. So the whole of the next chapter is dedicated to giving your liver the best possible food and using techniques to help it detoxify and help you reach optimum health and weight.

12.

L for Liver

The liver is the largest solid organ in your body, much bigger than most of us realize, sitting underneath the right lung and weighing in at 1.5 kilos (over 3 lb). Although the liver is very fragile, it can renew itself almost entirely. Amazingly, it can lose up to 90 per cent of its structure and still regenerate itself, given the right conditions, in just six weeks. It's an absolutely vital organ – it performs as many as 500 functions, many of them essential. The liver is the body's busiest filter, processor and metabolic factory. Everything that the body takes in (unless it's injected) passes through the liver, and every second of every day the liver is recycling and detoxifying to keep us healthy. If it's doing its job properly, the rest of the body works more efficiently and you'll be able to cleanse, lose weight and reach optimum health more easily. So we need to support this wonderful organ – our chemical factory – as much as possible during the 48-Hour Plan.

some of what the liver does:

Detoxifies – filters out and excretes waste and poisons – e.g. drugs, bacteria from our food. (The liver filters more than a litre of blood every minute!)

Manufactures bile.

Manufactures cholesterol.

Manufactures vitamin A and stores vitamins A, B12, D, E & K.

Manufactures enzymes.

Stores iron and copper.

Metabolizes carbohydrates, proteins and fats.

Disposes of dead blood cells.

Keeps immune system healthy and produces infection-fighting cells (such as microphages).

feeling 'liverish'

Liver stagnation and the need for detoxification usually come about through toxin or food excesses. If too much food is eaten, especially rich, greasy food, the liver becomes swollen and sluggish in an attempt to break it all down and dispose of it. Hence the expression 'liverish': a lovely old-fashioned word used to describe how people feel the day after eating and drinking too much! It's the same with alcohol, caffeine, drugs, high-protein diets, and exposure to external pollutants and chemicals. They all put too much strain on the liver, if consumed in large quantities.

TOP TIPS FOR HELPING THE LIVER THE MORNING AFTER THE NIGHT BEFORE

1. The best thing you can do for your liver is *undereat* – remember 'Give yourself permission *not* to eat'? If you're feeling 'liverish' you probably won't want to eat much anyway, so listen to your body and just drink plenty of water, and vegetable and fruit juices.

2. If you do feel like eating, make sure you eat plenty of fresh raw or steamed vegetables, especially those cruciferous vegetables such as broccoli, Brussels sprouts, cabbage, kale and cauliflower, because they're full of nutrients that really help the liver detox and unload.

3. Brown rice is considered *the* food of the liver in Chinese medicine, so make sure you have a small portion the morning after the night before, if you can eat.

4. Then have your *last* meal of that day in the afternoon so the liver and gall bladder have nothing else to do during their precious regeneration cycle from 11 p.m. to 3 a.m.

5. And don't have a hair of the dog! In fact, give up alcohol for a couple of days. This will help the liver to recover more quickly. Don't forget that 95 per cent of any alcohol drunk *has* to be metabolized in the liver, which means all the workers in the chemical factory will be so busy breaking down all those glasses of booze that they won't have time to do anything else. They won't manage to metabolize any fat that has been eaten, which means last night's packet of crisps or chips will just stay in the liver as a fatty build-up!

> **Remember, alcohol converts straight to fat, not to anything useful like glucose or glycogen.**

6. Don't take painkillers – they'll put an extra burden on the liver.

7. Do drink 'Liver Flush'. Mix the juice of half a lemon, half a clove of crushed garlic, a little grated fresh ginger and a dessertspoon of olive oil. Add a small glass of vegetable juice or vegetable stock, stir vigorously and drink. It sounds odd, but it does work – and the oil will help 'soak up' the alcohol.

carbs and the liver

The liver's health is also very important for the proper metabolizing of protein, fat and carbohydrate. Carbs – in the form of sugars and starches – are broken down by the digestion and absorbed into the bloodstream. The blood then travels to the liver, where the sugars are converted into glucose, the fuel the body needs for energy. A healthy liver regulates this fuel in the body and allows certain levels of glucose to circulate in the blood for the cells to use when they need it.

But if you eat *more* carbohydrate than is immediately required, the liver will convert that extra glucose into glycogen, which will be stored in the liver or in the muscles. Later on, when energy is needed, the liver will convert the glycogen back to glucose and return it to the bloodstream. *Excess* glucose is then converted into fatty acids and stored as body fat. The liver is very clever!

! TOP TIP FOR WEIGHT LOSS

If you regularly eat large quantities of carbs, however healthy they may be, and you don't exercise, you will put on weight. Body fat is simply a form of storage for energy. If you decrease your carbs intake and increase exercise those fat reserves are converted straight back to glucose for the body to use as fuel!

long-term liver imbalance

In Chinese medicine, the liver is recognized as being potentially the most congested of all the organs with too much fat and unmetabolized food and too many chemicals disrupting its valuable work and clogging it up. Traditional Chinese physiology states that a healthy liver establishes a smooth flow of energy (*chi*) through the whole person and that when the liver is 'happy' there is no stress or tension. People with unblocked healthy livers tend to be calm and happy, while people with a liver imbalance could be producing all sorts of physiological and psychological symptoms. Just check these lists to see if any of the signs ring a bell!

signs of a liver imbalance

EMOTIONAL

- Anger
- Impatience
- Frustration
- Resentment
- Rudeness
- Edginess
- Aggression
- Stubbornness
- Arrogance
- Violent Temper
- Mood Swings

PHYSICAL

- Nausea or Sickness
- Sudden, Explosive Bowel Movements
- Irregular or Heavy Periods
- Swollen Abdomen
- Migraines
- Craving for Oranges
- Pain that Moves around the Body
- Fibroids
- Cysts
- Haemorrhoids
- Eye Problems
- Red Cheeks

- Frequent Small Thirst
- Hot Palms and Soles of the Feet
- Insomnia

My take is that the liver is like the Planner, and if you treat the liver you're treating every other organ in your body, especially the kidneys and colon. If you suffer from constipation or a sluggish colon, looking after the liver and giving it everything you can to support it will, eventually, help your colon to function more efficiently. And don't forget, as you will see in chapter 15, you need your colon to be 'evacuating' as often as possible if those toxins are to leave your body!

Fasting or detoxing minimizes the liver's work – so the 48-Hour Plan will be like a three-day bank holiday weekend for this precious organ, giving it time to stop routine work and give itself a thorough spring clean! And the biggest help we can give the liver, apart from diet, is a technique as old as the hills!

castor oil packing for the liver

Castor oil was used therapeutically for hundreds, if not thousands, of years in ancient India, China, Persia, Egypt, Africa, Greece and Rome. Rather more recently, our grannies knew about the usefulness of castor oil and used it for all sorts of ailments before the advent of modern medicines. My grandmother used to make any child suffering from constipation swallow a tablespoon of castor oil. (Yuck!) What are less understood are the benefits of rubbing castor oil *into the skin* and how this can affect the nearest organs. One of my clients swears by it for relieving conditions as diverse as painful swollen toes and psoriasis.

benefits of castor oil packing

Improves colon elimination.
Reduces flatulence and nausea!
Improves digestive assimilation.
Stimulates liver, gall bladder and pancreas.
Improves lymphatic and blood circulations.
Draws acids and infections out of the body.
Reduces inflammation and swelling.
Relieves pain, including headaches.
Improves nervous system.

No one is too sure how castor oil works, but there are plenty of theories around, along with some scientific research. Applying castor oil to the skin, from where it is absorbed into the bloodstream, appears to act as a trigger for the prostaglandins – the potent hormone-like substances that affect blood pressure, metabolism, nerve impulses, immunity and, interestingly, inflammation. This could explain why my client's problems cleared up. Castor oil also seems to be 'bioenergetic', emitting a white light visible 6–8 inches around the container. Many complementary therapists believe that its extraordinary molecular make-up may have energetic properties similar to that of a *crystal*.

As far as the *liver* is concerned, the theory I like the most, and the one that has produced the best results for my clients and myself, is that putting castor oil on to the skin appears to release the mucus lying under the area where the oil is rubbed in. Don't ask me how or why, it just does! Your liver may have years' worth of toxicity in it, and castor oil packing can't possibly hurt you – it has to be worth a try, albeit a bit messy!

However, I am recommending castor oil packing for the liver only as part of a dedicated six-week or longer detox and not for the Weekend Plan. It's absolutely fine to regularly rub castor oil into the skin near an ache or pain, but using it on the liver with the packing method is a more serious undertaking. During a longer detox you should use the technique outlined below on three consecutive evenings a week, for three consecutive weeks. And then leave a week before repeating the regime. It would be a good idea to follow a three-day castor oil treatment with a colonic irrigation as your body needs to get all those backed-up toxins out as quickly as it possibly can. If you're doing a six-week detox, it might be worthwhile considering a colonic half way through your detox anyway to help shift things along! There's no point getting everything moving if it's got nowhere to go.

how to do castor oil packs

YOU WILL NEED:
Castor Oil
A Woollen or Normal Flannel
A Bin Liner, Plastic Bag (preferably without lettering – the castor oil might make this run) or Clingfilm
An Old Towel
A Hot-Water Bottle

METHOD:

Apply the castor oil generously to the flannel, but without saturating it.

Place over your liver.

Cover the flannel with a plastic food bag, or bin liner, or wrap clingfilm around the body to hold the cloth in place as it can leak and turn very messy.

Cover the whole area with an old towel, and wrap it around the body. A length of crêpe bandage can be used to hold it in place.

The hot-water bottle is then placed over the liver, to encourage the body to absorb the oil. Keep the hot-water bottle in place for 30–60 minutes while you rest, then remove it. You can then go to bed, leaving the oil on overnight.

Wash off the excess oil when you've finished, or the next morning.

Store the cloth in an airtight container. It can be reused lots of times before it needs washing.

THE LAZY, QUICK WAY – ALMOST AS EFFECTIVE!

Cover the skin above the liver in castor oil, and sit in a warm (not hot) bath for a minimum of 20 minutes. After that, you can either leave the oil on and wear an old T-shirt, or wash it off and go to bed. Either way, your skin will have absorbed most of it and you will sleep like a log.

Or: Cover the area over the liver in castor oil, put a filthy old T-shirt on, place a hot-water bottle on top, and go to bed. Remove the hot-water bottle after 30–60 minutes and go to sleep.

Again, this can be done on three nights in a row per week for three consecutive weeks. Then have a week off before repeating.

For the Weekend Plan, I'm suggesting an Epsom salts bath (explained in chapter 15). These don't work on the liver to quite the same degree as castor oil packing, but they do a very good job getting the lymph moving and detoxifying you, and are hugely relaxing.

13. I for **Integration**

Integration means looking at more techniques to incorporate into your 48-Hour Plan, and into the rest of your life, that will help balance you in body, mind and spirit and get those stress levels right down. Today, more than ever, we suffer from tension, stress and the 'too much to do' syndrome. Millions of us in the UK alone are turning to tranquillizers, sleeping pills and alcohol to relax us, and one in three of us will go to a doctor at some point in our lives suffering from depression. A recent report issued by the European Commission cited stress as the second most common health problem after back pain: 41.2 million people in the EU were affected in 2000 – that's more than the entire population of Spain!

We've looked at diet in depth, and the exercises suggested in chapter 10 will help us by releasing those 'natural high' hormones – endorphins. The yoga will work on another level by stimulating all our internal organs and calming our mind. But if we are to get our stress levels way down and fine-tune every cell in the body, we need to incorporate some of the following suggestions into our daily routine. Think of these techniques as the valeting after your car has gone through its MOT!

integration techniques

Tibetan Twirling
Tongue-Scraping
Teeth-Cleaning

Simple Breathing –
    Pranayama
Simple Relaxation
Simple Meditation

Have a read through and decide which suggestions appeal to you so you can try some of them out *before* the Plan. There are only 6 techniques and they are all worth trying to build into your daily routine even though, like me, you'll probably convince yourself you just don't have enough time! When I do get back into the daily habit of kicking off the day with some simple yoga movements, followed by the integration techniques, the day seems to flow along effortlessly, nothing stresses me and I feel and look more energized and positive. So I can only urge you at least to give them a go during the Weekend, when you *will* have all the time you need. Once you're back in the real world they can take as little time as 30 seconds to 5 minutes each, much like brushing your teeth. It's simply a question of getting into the habit and deciding which ones you're going to do – every day, no matter what!

tibetan twirling

This exercise is going to make you feel like a mad whirling Dervish! It's not only fun but has hidden health benefits as well. This is one exercise that you can always make time for at the beginning of your day as it's really speedy and will wake up your whole system.

According to the Tibetan lamas, and many Ayurvedic practitioners, there are seven energy vortexes in the body centred on our seven endocrine glands: the reproductive glands, the pancreas, the adrenals, the thymus, the thyroid gland, the pineal gland and the pituitary gland. These glands make our hormones and send them out into the bloodstream to be carried to all our organs and tissues for every body function. According to the philosophy, if one of the glands slows down because of ageing or ill health, the flow of *prana* – the life force that in Ayurvedic medicine means 'vital breath' – also slows down and dis-ease may set in.

One of the quickest ways to get that *prana* moving is by spinning. When all the vortexes revolve at great speed and at the *same* speed the body is in perfect health!

how to spin

Find a nice big space, where you're not going to stumble into any furniture, and where the floor is not slippery. (Maybe try the garden patio.)

Stand up straight with your arms stretched out, parallel to the floor, and spin round clockwise until you become dizzy – it usually takes 5–6 times. Keep practising till you have built up to 20 revolutions, maybe increasing by one every couple of days. Make sure your feet are squarely on the ground throughout, and spin as fast as you can without falling over!

To help combat dizziness, you could try the trick that dancers and skaters use. Fix your eyes on an object or a mark on the wall in front of you, level with your eyes, and keep your eyes on that point for as long as possible while you're turning. Your head will have to keep up with your body, but turn your head at the last possible moment really quickly so you can stare at the same spot as you come round. But be careful not to hurt your neck by moving it too quickly!

Spinning regularly as a technique for a healthier, stress-free life sounds mad, I know, but at the very worst it'll wake you up and get all those cells buzzing. And at best you'll be healthier and calmer. The Hale Clinic's Ayurvedic Doctor, Doja Purkit, recommends that we all practise spinning if we want a tension-free day: 'If you can spin 20 times you will never feel stress,' he says. Dr Purkit believes spinning replicates the turbulence caused by stress in the body's cells, which will help the body to understand and overcome it.

Whatever spinning does (and it seems to work for me), it's fun, it's free and it's something the whole family can enjoy – so give it a whirl!

tongue-scraping and teeth-cleaning

Are you old enough to remember when GPs used to look at your tongue to gauge your internal health? Doctors don't seem to do this any more, but *we* can. By having a quick look at your tongue every morning, before you clean your teeth, you'll be able to see how your digestion is doing. If you also get into a daily habit of *scraping* your tongue you'll be sending a wake-up call to your gastric juices. As soon as the millions of taste buds on your tongue are stimulated they send a message to the digestive system to get ready and your food will be broken down more efficiently.

Studying and scraping my tongue every morning is, to me, as important as cleaning my teeth. Let's face it, teeth don't change much in appearance from day to day. But the tongue does. How coated is it? How white? Does your breath smell?

If there is a thick white coating on the tongue, it means there is a lot of toxicity in the system, from a heavy or too late meal the night before. It could be that you're still digesting last evening's food, in which case a very light breakfast or just a juice would be the best thing to give your digestion a rest. Or it may be that all that de-toxing over the Weekend is coming out of your system and showing on your tongue, giving it a nice white, furred appearance!

To scrape the tongue, use a tongue scraper (sold in health shops or by mail order) or a small spoon. Gently move from the back of the tongue forward until you have scraped the entire surface. The whole process only takes 20 seconds and will get rid of that unpleasant coating, clear bacteria out of your mouth and make your breath smell sweeter!

teeth-cleaning

There are two quick tips for healthier teeth. The first suggestion, I must admit, isn't one I have time for every day, but is well worth doing during a weekend off. The second one is quick, simple and *can* be done every day after cleaning your teeth.

Massage your gums: According to Eastern medicine, you can make your teeth healthier and more beautiful by massaging your gums daily. Take a mouthful of warm sesame oil and swish it from side to side for 2–3 minutes. Don't swallow it. Spit out the oil, then massage your gums with your index finger. This is, apparently, brilliant for preventing receding gums, tooth infections and cavities.

Tap your teeth: Tap your teeth together 5 or 6 times gently (so you don't disturb any crowns or fillings!). This is said to stimulate the energy meridians related to the teeth. Again, this should get that *prana* moving and wake up all your organs.

simple breathing – *pranayama*

benefits of pranayama

Expels stress and relaxes you.
Stills the mind.
Works as a quick meditation.
Increases mental clarity.

Increase oxygen supply.
Improves digestion.
Recharges the batteries.
Increases physical energy.

Pranayama is a very useful detoxing aid because *breathing deeply expels 70 per cent of the toxins in the body*. But the most important reason to do pranayama, I believe, is because of its effect on the brain. We know that there are two hemispheres in the brain with different functions: the left for logic, languages and figures and the right for creativity, imagination and intuition. By alternating the nostrils (as you will see in a minute) you are sending the breath to each side of the brain in turn, which will help balance the two hemispheres. It's known as a neuromuscular integration, which basically means that you're merging mind and body and creating greater mental clarity and energy.

We do it at the end of yoga classes and it always makes me feel much sharper, more focused and relaxed. More importantly, doing it in the morning really seems to help me with any mental tasks, especially if I'm doing it outdoors in the fresh air.

Because you have to concentrate quite hard on doing these exercises properly, they also give you a chance for a bit of 'quiet' time. Even if the only time you have is sitting on the loo in the morning they're nearly as beneficial as a quick meditation and only take five minutes.

how to do *Pranayama*

Sit comfortably with your spine as straight as possible.

Close your eyes and rest your left hand on your knee – you'll be using your right hand.

Keep your mouth shut throughout.

Using your right thumb, close off your right nostril. Then, through your left nostril, inhale slowly and deeply. Hold the breath for four counts.

Now with your middle fingers close your left nostril and exhale slowly out of your right nostril.

Then, keeping your left nostril closed, inhale through your right nostril, and hold the breath for four counts.

Move your thumb on to your right nostril and exhale through the left nostril.

Repeat the sequence using alternate nostrils for about 5 minutes.

Your breathing may be slightly slower and deeper than usual, but it should be natural and unforced.

When you're finished, just sit quietly for a few minutes and breathe normally.

simple relaxation

The body is cooled down and stilled by complete relaxation, which eases tension in the muscles and rests the whole system, leaving you as refreshed as after a good night's sleep. Relaxation carries over into all your activities and teaches you to conserve your energy and let go of worries and fears. This technique also serves as a great pick-me-up if you're going out straight after work and feel exhausted. It helps you relax in bed at night if you're having trouble sleeping. And, most importantly during the Plan, it's an excellent technique to do after meals to prevent you from rushing around when you should be relaxing and digesting.

My lovely yoga teacher Patricia Haygarth came up with this wonderful relaxation exercise, which is the final relaxation after a yoga session. You can do it at any time of the day or night. You can spend five minutes on it, or much longer if you like.

Lie flat on your back with your feet apart, the toes rolling away from the heels. Your arms are at your sides and slightly away from the body, with the palms facing up. Make sure your head is straight and your neck is long. Allow your mind to help the body relax and repeat mentally to yourself as you travel through the body, beginning with your toes, 'I relax my toes . . . my toes are relaxed. I relax my feet and ankles . . . my feet and ankles are relaxed. I relax my legs . . . my legs are relaxed. I relax my hips . . . my tummy . . . my arms . . . my chest . . . my back . . . my neck . . . my face . . .' until you reach your head and finally your mind. *Relax. Relax. Relax.*

simple meditation

Meditation has been shown to boost the immune system, calm the mind, get rid of negative thoughts and even fight disease. Millions of people around the world swear by it, but you don't need to sit cross-legged on the floor, chanting, for three hours a day in order to meditate properly and reap the benefits.

The whole point of meditation is to still the brain, to visualize thoughts plopping into your mind, but to ignore them and let them drift out again. The more you practise meditation the quieter your thoughts will become – it's almost like telling your mind to 'shut up'. Doing meditation regularly will help reduce stress and fatigue and will really improve your energy levels and make you feel happy and calm. Set aside five minutes when you won't be interrupted, twice a day. Even these short sessions will have a beneficial effect. But, during the 48-Hour Plan, try to spend longer on meditation. Twenty minutes – twice a day – would be really good for you!

how to meditate

Use a quiet room away from traffic noise, children noise and other distractions, even if it's just the bathroom. (Use earplugs if there's too much noise.) Make sure you're wearing warm and comfortable clothes. Take your shoes off and sit cross-legged on the floor or, if you have trouble keeping your spine straight, sit with your back against a wall. Or sit on a chair, as long as it's straight-backed and your feet are resting comfortably on the floor. (Or even lie down – I don't recommend this as I always fall asleep!) Sit with your palms up and open like empty bowls, resting on your knees.

Close your eyes. Keep them relaxed and imagine there is a white dot between your eyebrows. Breathe normally, but as you inhale and exhale, gradually begin to notice your breathing. Don't try and influence your breathing in any way, just follow it. Allow it to reach its own rhythm.

If your brain starts getting busy and making lists, don't try to stop it. Look at each thought, imagine it in a bubble and just blow it away. Then come back to following your breathing. It's a very simple exercise but it takes a little practice to get used to 'watching' those thoughts, letting go of them, and getting back into stillness and nothingness.

so-hum meditation

Abid Dar, my acupuncturist, taught me this meditation to help me overcome my Busy Brain Syndrome, and it works for me.

So if you have a real problem letting go of those thoughts, try this. In So-Hum meditation we sit quietly and follow our breathing as before, but we add the sound *So* on inhalation and *Hum* on exhalation. Don't say the sounds out loud – say them to yourself. You'll be much more focused.

Hum means 'I' or 'individual ego'; *So* means 'He, the Divine'. When *So* goes in, life energy also goes in, and when *Hum* goes out, our ego also goes out. That's the significance of So-Hum meditation.

At the end of your meditation, just sit quietly and let your body come back to the present. You'll feel so relaxed and energized you'll wonder why you've never done it before! Again, it's a wonderful technique to use if you come in from work exhausted, wondering how you're going to keep going through the evening. Try it for just five minutes!

! TOP TIP – TREE ENERGY

Believe it or not, sitting cross-legged under a tree, making sure your back is in contact with the trunk, has an energizing effect. If you don't have time for the breathing or meditation exercises, try this instead for 5 minutes and see how 'grounded' and calm you feel! People always make fun of hippies who hug trees, but I really do think there's something in it. If you believe, as I do, that all 'life' on this planet is linked in some way, then the life force and energy that is contained in a 200-year-old tree must have *some* effect on us at a cellular level. Try it during the 48-Hour Plan – you've nothing to lose, although you might get some strange looks from passers-by!

14. F for **Fats:** The Essential Ones

Because we've come to associate *all* fats with bad health, patients usually have a fit when I start cajoling them to eat more essential fats – they think they're going to put on weight. But I'm not talking here about *saturated* fats in foods such as *cheese*, *coconut*, *lard*, *suet*, *bacon* and *fatty meats*. We all know they go straight to our thighs and are bad for our heart if eaten in excess. *Hydrogenated* fats such as *margarines* aren't the right kind of fats either because they're *trans-fatty acids*, which new studies have shown to be even worse for long-term health than saturated fats. I'm talking about essential fatty acids (EFAs) and, actually, you can't possibly lose weight effectively *without* them because of their fantastic effect on your metabolism.

3 reasons why efas are not fattening

1. EFAs help you reach your ideal weight because they increase your metabolic rate and speed up the transfer of oxygen to the cells. Fuel is burnt more efficiently.

2. Your body needs every bit of these precious fats for all the jobs they do, so it's hardly going to waste them and store them as fat – they're far too valuable.

3. These oils are a bit like the doormen of the cells. They help to open the cells to let the sodium out – remember the electrolyte balance? So if you want your body to release toxicity that's locked in the cells, and therefore some of the excess weight, you need the oils to open the gates.

And, more importantly, EFAs have such a dramatic and immediate impact on energy, stress and hormone levels that once you start taking them regularly you'll never be without them again, you'll feel so good. Our bodies cannot manufacture EFAs; we have to rely on our food to supply us with the right amounts. The two EFAs that our body needs to convert into something it can use are linoleic (Omega 6) and linolenic (Omega 3) acids. Generally, Omega 6 isn't an EFA we are short of in our diet. We *are*, however, extremely short of Omega 3, so during the Plan we will make sure we're boosting our intake of this useful fat.

more benefits of efas

Help foetal development: A foetus needs fatty acids for brain development, eye, cell, skin and joint health, and liver function. And it has been found that mothers who consume more oily fish or fish-oil capsules during pregnancy produce healthier, brighter children.

Brain health: EFAs, especially Omega 3, are essential for the brain, because nearly a *quarter* of the brain's structure is made up of fatty acids. Having them in the body in the right quantities helps memory and concentration and reduces depression.

I believe that one cause of post-natal depression may be that the foetus takes much-needed Omega 3 for its own development out of the mother's blood. If the mother isn't eating enough Omega 3 to compensate for this, she may end up so deficient in EFAs in her own brain that she will suffer from depression.

EFAs have also been shown to help in the treatment of behavioural problems in children, including hyperactivity.

Help the central nervous system: EFAs are needed for healthy cell membranes, especially in the nerve cells.

Good for the heart and blood circulation: Omega 3 has been shown to lower cholesterol levels and blood pressure, and prevent hardening of the arteries. After a heart attack, eating oily fish three times a week halves the risk of having another attack.

Good for your skin, nails and hair: EFAs are natural moisturizers. Without them the cells are unable to hold on to water and the skin and scalp will become dry and flaky, and the nails brittle.

Boost immunity: EFAs strengthen the immunity by building up the good bacteria in the intestines and by giving the cells more energy to remove waste and fight viruses and harmful bacteria.

Reduce inflammation: Omega 3 helps produce anti-inflammatory chemicals (those useful prostaglandins).

Improve bowel and digestive functions: I have seen such success with patients suffering from all manner of bowel problems – from diverticulosis to constipation – that I just want to shout this one out from the rooftops! Plenty of Omega 3, in the form of linseed oil, really works.

Helps the hormonal balance: Linseeds (rich in Omega 3) are full of phytoestrogens, which mimic natural oestrogen and help level out the hormones. Evening primrose, blackcurrant-seed and starflower oil (rich in Omega 6), are also extremely helpful with balancing hormones, and especially with mitigating PMS symptoms such as lumpy breasts.

Help process and distribute fat-soluble vitamins: EFAs are vital if the fat-soluble vitamins – A, D, E and K – are to be taken up by the body. Vitamin E is used as an antioxidant, A (beta-carotene) promotes healthy eyes and membranes, D aids in calcium absorption and K is needed for blood-clotting and preventing bleeding.

Help you beat those winter blues! Omega 3 is known as 'antifreeze' because it keeps the blood thin and circulating in cold weather. Enough Omega 3 in your diet will keep your hands and feet warm in the winter, and you won't even notice the lack of sunlight, so you won't fall prey to SAD.

As we've already noted, our modern diet deprives us of the right balance of the two EFAs. So let's look at what we should be eating.

efa sources

TYPE OF EFA	SOURCES
Linoleic Acid (Omega 6)	Nuts, Sunflower, Pumpkin & Sesame Seeds, Grains, Pulses, Vegetables and Fruit
converted in the body to	
GLA	Breast Milk, Spirulina, Evening Primrose Oil, Blackcurrant and Borage (Starflower) Seeds
Linolenic Acid (Omega 3)	Linseeds, Pumpkin Seeds, Walnuts and Dark Green Vegetables
converted in the body to	
EPA & DHA	Cold-Water Oily Fish, such as Salmon, Sardines, Tuna, Mackerel and Herring

(I won't complicate things too much by explaining exactly what GLA, EPA and DHA are – but note that they are *conversion products* of Omega 3 and 6.)

For our body functions, we do need a steady intake of Omega 6. But today we consume far too much of this in relation to Omega 3, something like 20 times too much. The ideal ratio should be no less than 1 part Omega 6 to 1 part Omega 3, and no more than 5:1. But because our consumption of oily fish has declined by a staggering 80 per cent in the last 100 years, that ratio is all out of kilter. As you'll be getting more than enough Omega 6 from the Plan's suggestions, we'll be concentrating this Weekend on the EFA that's most lacking, Omega 3, in plant form.

omega 3

Omega 3 fatty acids help to produce a type of prostaglandin (3 series) which has been shown to:

Reduce the inflammation caused by arthritis.

Relax blood vessels.

Lower blood pressure.

Reduce the stickiness of blood.

Improve cholesterol levels.

Play an important role in hormone production.

Influence metabolism.

Affect nerve transmission and gut function.

The richest source of Omega 3 is found in *linseeds* (flaxseeds) and *linseed* (flaxseed) *oil* – and, no, I don't mean the stuff your partner or dad puts on his cricket bat! Linseed oil is even more potent than fish oil (and it's also a good source of Omega 6).

The other good source of Omega 3 is cold-water oily fish such as salmon, sardines and mackerel. Fresh tuna is also an excellent source – but tinned won't provide as much (unless you drizzle linseed oil over it!). Cod itself is low in EFAs, but cod-liver oil is one of the richest sources of Omega 3 – the trouble is, it's also one of the most concentrated sources of any toxins that are in the fish livers. This is why I tend to encourage patients who can't eat or don't like fish itself or linseed oil to supplement their diets with fish oils (EPA – eicosapentaenoic acid) made from the bodies of oily fish rather than cod livers.

As you can see from the sources diagram, there is a difference in the way the body can absorb fish oils, compared to the way it uses linseeds and linseed oil. If you eat fish or take fish oils, you're saving the body from having to do a conversion. For some this may be beneficial: babies can't do the conversion, nor can the elderly or the very sick. So if you come into any of these categories, or are pregnant, fish oils in capsule form (EPA) will be better for you than linseed oil.

You might be sitting there thinking, Why bother with the linseed oil if I can get all the benefits from oily fish? To provide the required amount of Omega 3 you would need to eat a portion of salmon at least three times a week. And how many of us have either the time or the budget? Besides, many readers are vegetarians or vegans, who won't even consider taking fish oil capsules.

More importantly, because the 48-Hour Plan is focusing on 'plant' food and cleansing, linseeds and linseed oil are top of the menu because they will give you a huge boost of the much-needed Omega 3 fats without contributing any acidity. I'm trying to make this plan as supplement-free as possible, and this is the quickest and simplest way of getting Omega 3 (and 6) in the right proportions into your body on a daily basis.

In case you're still wondering whether EFAs are a good idea, look at the checklist below to see whether a significant number of these health problems apply to you.

symptoms of omega 3 & 6 deficiency checklist

- Dry Skin or other Skin Problems
- Poor Nails and Hair
- Low Metabolism
- Tired all the time
- Depression
- Post-Natal Depression
- Poor Memory
- High Blood Pressure
- High Cholesterol Levels
- Varicose Veins
- Arthritis

- Aching Joints
- Inflammation
- Infertility
- Hormone Fluctuation
- PMS
- Lumpy Breasts
- Water Retention
- Bowel Problems
- Gallstones
- Seasonal Affective Disorder – SAD
- Blood-Sugar Blues

efa daily regime for the plan

You'll be starting the day off with a fabulous smoothie to get just the right amount of EFAs into your system. You'll be using linseeds, linseed oil and lecithin granules in the following quantities:

1. linseeds/flaxseeds: 1 tablespoon

Whole linseeds are a rich source of fibre, minerals and protein as well as of essential fats. They are also full of phytoestrogens, which we know help with hormone levels. And, whether you're constipated or not, they will really help drag those toxins out of your colon during the 48-Hour Plan.

Aim to have *1 tablespoon of soaked linseeds (flaxseeds) per day*. Put a tablespoon of golden linseeds in a glass last thing the night before and, because they will swell quite a bit, add plenty of water to more than cover them. The seeds are full of zinc and vitamin E, as well as Omega 3, so none of that goodness is wasted if you use the water along with the seeds. In the morning the seeds will be soft and gelatinous, so they won't rush through your intestines scraping them, but go through very slowly and gently, cleaning your colon like a broom.

One of my elderly clients had suffered from chronic constipation for five years and would be in such pain by the third day that she would be forced to use laxatives. After just four days of eating soaked linseeds, she started going to the loo, naturally, every morning for the first time in years. Another one had not had a regular bowel movement since giving up cigarettes. Her body missed the nicotine trigger! She too says the soaked linseeds changed her life — and her bowels — for ever.

2. linseed oil: 1–2 tablespoons

Make sure you buy a good-quality linseed oil that is cold-pressed and sold in a dark glass bottle. Oils oxidize very easily and can go rancid, so keep the bottle in the fridge. DO NOT HEAT UP THE OIL.

You may find linseed oil to be an acquired taste, or you may love it! If you hate it, don't panic, because once it's mixed with the rest of the smoothie ingredients, especially the lecithin granules, you won't know it's there. But if you like it, which I hope you will, you can also use it for salad dressings or drizzle it over your cooked meal *once the food has been taken off the heat.*

3. lecithin granules: 1 teaspoon–1 tablespoon

Lecithin is a nutrient and an oil found in most living tissues — particularly in those covering the brain and nerve cells — and is therefore pretty important for your body's health. Lecithin forms part of the cell membrane and plays an essential part in helping movement in and out of the cells.

Lecithin is very rich in Omega 6, which will balance the Omega 3 in the linseed oil, and is very useful for protecting and regenerating the liver. Because of its high vitamin B content, it's also excellent for the brain, the memory and for hangovers! That should be enough of an incentive to add it to your smoothie!

Commercially, lecithin is extracted from eggs, soya beans or corn, so if you are a strict vegetarian check the ingredients to make sure of its source. You might also want to check that the soya isn't genetically modified.

When you put the lecithin granules into the smoothie they emulsify the linseed oil so the whole thing turns into a creamy, milkshake-like drink with no trace of any oil. Start with a teaspoon of lecithin granules and build up to a tablespoon, if you like it and feel good on it. Some people need time for their livers to adjust, while others love it straight off. Just listen to your body and see how it reacts.

suzi's smoothie recipe

Ingredients:

1 apple or pear
1 kiwi fruit
2–3 strawberries, plus a few blackberries, blueberries
    or raspberries – any berries, including frozen
    ones
1 teaspoon–1 tablespoon of lecithin granules
1–2 tablespoons of linseed oil
1 tablespoon of soaked linseeds with the water
1 handful of ground pumpkin and sunflower seeds
2–4 almonds
1 brazil nut
Cranberry, apple or any fruit juice if you need more liquid
1 tablespoon of aloe vera juice (optional)

Put these ingredients in the blender, whizz them up and drink! If the smoothie isn't sweet enough, you might like to add acouple of dates, or a spoonful of honey. You may prefer to try other fruits but these work for me. I particularly like the berries because they make the smoothie taste like a creamy, berry milkshake – without the milk!

You'll find this smoothie incredibly filling and it should keep you going for hours – perfect for a detoxing weekend, or a nutritious, energizing breakfast.

15.

E for **Exit Routes**

During your Weekend, you'll need to use all the exit routes your body has in order to cleanse the toxicity out of your system. Again, I marvel at how clever the body actually is because, in naturopathic terms, a healthy body stays healthy by cleansing continuously to keep its cell membranes fluid and in good condition. Fortunately, we have all these holes just waiting to discharge toxins and waste out of the body! But they need a little help.

The body will often resort to a route that it has used before. If you're someone who has suffered from catarrh all your life, that's the route the body will default to. If you get cold sores when run down – guess what – the body will produce more cold sores if it needs to move toxins out of your body quickly. These healing crises are very boring – but they *are* part of the healing process. You often get worse before you get better. But you *will* get better and stronger and, once you have detoxified, may find chronic conditions that have plagued you all your life will finally disappear for good.

the body's exit routes

Eyes	Skin
Nose	Colon
Ears	Uterus
Lungs and Mouth	Kidneys

eyes

Hopefully, you won't be weeping or developing conjunctivitis over the Weekend! But it's worth noting that if you *do* feel tearful and want a good cry for no reason, then go ahead and have one, and justify your temporary insanity by accepting that crying is a good way of getting stuff out! Have you noticed how much better you always feel after a good cry! I'm convinced that those tears are not only releasing emotional toxins that need to be eliminated, but also some of the physical toxins accumulated along the way. We now know that letting go of emotions is incredibly important for a healthy immune system – so go on, let it out. Better out than in!

nose

If you get a cold while you're cleansing, welcome it and think of it as another route your body is using. The more mucus-inducing your diet was before starting the programme (lots of dairy products, chocolate, pasta, etc.) the more mucus has to come out once you've made changes.

Should you go down with the sniffles, rest as much as you need to, drink as much liquid as you can, try not to take any suppressants and give your body time. The quickest way to heal is to rest and eat as little as possible, so that your body concentrates on fighting the virus. But if you're anything like me, you'll have an enormous appetite and will want to 'feed your cold'. In that case, go with the flow and eat as often as you like, especially immunity-boosting foods such as fruit and veg. As tempting as 'comfort foods' are, remember that even a small sugar intake can reduce your immunity by up to half.

! TOP TIPS FOR TREATING A COLD

Keep warm.
Rest.
Drink lots of hot water with honey & lemon.
Try the hydrotherapy suggestions in chapter 8.
Inhale the steam from elderflower teabags infusing in a bowl of hot water – as good as Vick's inhaler! Or try Olbas, a brilliant natural decongestant.
Try not to keep blowing your nose, it's better to spit!
Take a vitamin C with zinc supplement.

WARNING: Large doses of vitamin C can cause a very loose tummy – if that's the case, reduce the dosage or stay near a loo. If you're on any medication or have a history of kidney complaints consult your doctor before taking vitamin C supplements.

Take echinacea herbal tincture for 10 days (but not longer, and use as directed).
Put warming spices in your food such as ginger, cayenne pepper, chillies and garlic.

ears

I really hope nothing starts coming out of your ears during the detox! But if you do find that you have any ear problems or have a build-up of wax heavier than normal, assume that your body has found another weakness and exit route to use. Chronic ear problems are associated with an over-consumption of *wheat*, *milk*, *corn*, *eggs*, *yeast*, *soya* and *sugar*. Your new diet will lessen your chances of suffering from frequent ear problems.

lungs and mouth

If you get a really chesty cough, which is considered by naturopaths to be a form of cleansing rather than a weakness, get the phlegm moving out of your lungs by inhaling deeply to loosen it. And then, in the privacy of your bathroom, *spit out* as much of the disgusting stuff as possible! Recently I was suffering from the end of a streaming cold/cleanse and just happened to be working with a group of GPs. One of them told me that spitting is much better for you than blowing your nose as it encourages the debris to exit more rapidly and easily, and the virus doesn't hang around in your body. I was a bit taken aback – I certainly wasn't going to start spitting in the middle of a meeting! But it's worth thinking about.

cough cures

Again, none of the over-the-counter cough medicines seem to work, do they? Even doctors and pharmacists now say you're better off having an ordinary hot drink or sucking a boiled sweet, and saving your money. The best drink in my book is *hot water with lemon, honey, grated ginger and a bit of brandy or Scotch*! Not ideal for a detox – but better than a suppressant and at least you'll sleep. You could try rubbing castor oil on your chest (see chapter 12 – that could really help to shift some of that phlegm).

mouth ulcers

If you get mouth ulcers during a detox, it's a sodium (or sugar) release. Basically, there's too much acidity in your system and it's trying to get out.

> **! TOP TIP** FOR MOUTH ULCERS
>
> Gargle with black tea as it has antibacterial properties. Add a dash of lemon because that's a mild antiseptic.

cold sores

Some people suffer from an outbreak of cold sores when they get into a deep cleanse – and I used to be one of those people. It's very common amongst those of us who love salty foods rather than sweet foods. In fact, anything on the skin that is sore, burning or itching is usually a sign of a very high sodium level in the body. Remember that sodium/calcium balance? However, I hardly ever suffer from then now because my diet and EFA balance are right, keeping cold sores at bay.

Personally, I don't go along with the theory that nuts bring on attacks of cold sores because of their high content of the amino acid arginine. I eat loads of nuts! Many practitioners recommend taking the beneficial amino acid supplement Lysine to help *prevent* frequent attacks, but I rely on my diet.

If you do get the slightest warning or tingling over the Weekend, don't buy over-the-counter remedies. In my experience, they suppress a sore so that it comes back in another place later. A far more natural treatment is lemon balm (melissa) essential oil, which has been found to block the nerve cells that the virus normally infects. If used early enough it's supposed to get rid of a cold sore in as little as four hours – and I'm happy to back that up because it has certainly worked that quickly for me. Apart from the wonderful melissa, rest and drink as much fluid as you can, and boost your immune system by following the Plan for longer than 48 hours.

! **TOP TIPS** FOR COLD SORES

Frequently dab on melissa – in cream, tincture or oil form – at the first sign of an outbreak.
A diet high in zinc may aid prevention: eat oysters and pumpkin seeds.
A diet high in lecithin and EFAs will certainly keep them at bay.
Echinacea tincture taken for 10 days will boost immunity.

---

skin

As you already know, from reading about the lymph system, the skin is our largest organ and the body's largest exit route, which needs to be used for excreting salts, toxins and metabolic wastes as much as possible over the Weekend. You may suffer from a worse than usual outbreak of spots, rashes or eczema while you're detoxing – again this is your body getting a little worse before it gets better.

We have already covered skin-brushing in depth to help eliminate the waste gathering in the lymph and on the outside of the skin. But we can also increase the skin's ability to excrete by *sweating* as much as possible.

steams and saunas

Steams and saunas have been used for thousands of years to open the skin's pores and cleanse the body. Saunas are a very *dry* heat, like in the desert, and steam rooms produce a very *moist* heat, like in a rainforest. Whichever you prefer, they'll both make the sweat pour off you in a very short session.

You don't need to join an expensive health club to enjoy the benefits of a sauna or steam. Some public swimming pools have them, and they are very reasonably priced. There are always clear instructions on using the facilities, and check with your doctor if in any doubt about taking a steam or sauna. If you haven't tried one before, start with only a couple of minutes and build up the sessions to five minutes or longer. Some people have a cold shower and then go in for a second stint. If you can't take the shock of cold water, make it a cool-to-warm shower instead. Always end on a coolish shower.

If you can't get to a steam room or sauna, don't worry – you can do your own version at home, and for free!

MAKING A STEAM ROOM IN YOUR BATHROOM

Make sure there are no gaps around the window, turn the shower on to the hottest temperature and close the bathroom door behind you. Roll up a towel and put it along the bottom of the door, so no hot air can escape. Leave the shower running for a good 10 minutes. This will fill the bathroom with steam (and is also a great tip if you're ever stuck in a hotel with a creased outfit and no iron!).

Once the bathroom is hot and steamy, go and sit in there and sweat (move the towel to the inside of the door). You won't sweat buckets like you would in a steam room, but it's not a bad alternative for cleansing the skin.

Another option is a lovely warm/hot bath. The best bath for detoxing purposes has to be an Epsom salts bath, because it encourages the skin to release toxins.

detoxing bath for the weekend: epsom salts bath

Epsom salts are magnesium sulphate. As you'll remember, magnesium is one of the minerals we want to get back *into* the cells to improve the electrolyte balance. Magnesium also relaxes the muscles. Soaking in an Epsom salts bath will *increase sweating* and help any muscular aches and pains you might have. It's very good for people suffering from arthritis or sciatica and will help fight colds, flu and other viruses.

The temperature should be as hot as is comfortable. Add 1 cup of Epsom salts to a full bath and soak in it for 10–20 minutes. Do this on three consecutive evenings over the Plan Weekend. After the bath, wrap up warmly, drink plenty of water and rest. You'll sleep like a baby after one of these sessions!

If you're on a longer detox, you can have this bath on three consecutive evenings per week for three weeks. Then leave a week before repeating.

colon

The colon may not be the *largest* organ of toxin elimination, but it's the most *important*. Like many other practitioners, I believe a healthy colon means a healthy body and the first sign of dis-ease usually starts there with severe dehydration and constipation caused by stress, poor nutrition and a lack of fluid. Don't forget the colon needs masses of water to help push waste through.

why colon health is important for the whole health of a person

The digestive tract is one long tube from mouth to anus – food goes in at the top and waste comes out at the end. The upper part of the system (mouth, stomach and small intestine) is designed for *absorption*, the lower part (large intestine, including the colon) for *elimination*.

The colon is about six feet long and should be about two inches in diameter. We all should have more than a kilo (2 lb) of *friendly* bacteria living in harmony with our body. They're provided with a home and regular meals and in return break down the fibre and waste in the colon to get it moving out. But not all bacteria are as useful, and if someone has consumed fast food, meat, milk, sugar, booze and repeated courses of antibiotics for too long the unfriendly bacteria will multiply like mad and produce toxins, wind and bloating.

After years of poor diet, the colon may be full of mucoid plaque, the friendly bacteria will have been killed off, and the colon's peristalsis will have slowed down. A dehydrated and sluggish colon will not eliminate waste from the body efficiently.

I consider it healthy to go to the loo once or, preferably, twice a day. Food transit time through the system should be less than 24 hours, so that no more than two or three meals are in the gut at a time. Today's lunch should be pushing out yesterday's dinner, so that nothing is hanging around festering. The trouble is, many people think it's completely normal not to go to the loo every day, and only go every couple of days, storing several days' worth of meals in a very bloated gut. I used to think that those huge abdomens you see on some men were just beer bellies. Now I know better; they're carrying around masses of putrefying food and bacteria in their colon, as much as 20 lb of it!

However, a diet high in fruit, vegetables, oils, seeds, brown rice *and water* will encourage your bowel to do what it's supposed to do – get rid of waste twice a day.

! TOP TIP – PSYLLIUM HUSKS

You may want to try psyllium husks, which are a safe herbal laxative. They will help the bowel wall to push bulk along smoothly and quickly, with no straining or pain, and they stimulate the friendly bacteria in the bowel. Psyllium husks are a good source of fibre (much better than bran, which can often make matters worse) and they can absorb many times their own weight in fluid, removing unwanted, impacted waste from the colon walls. Mixed

> with water they can taste like sawdust, so try this: stir
> 1–2 teaspoons of psyllium husks into a little *apple or*
> *cranberry juice* and leave to soak for a few hours or
> overnight in a suitable container, such as a small glass.
> You'll end up with a mini jelly – much nicer!

what does the perfect stool look like?

We're very embarrassed about our bowel habits in the UK, unlike other countries such as Germany, where it's completely normal to look at your poos before flushing them away. (They even have shelves built into their toilets to help them study them!) 'What do they look like?' is a question that never fails to make my patients really uncomfortable. However, if you want a healthy body and bowel, then I'm afraid you need to get used to having a quick peek at your poos to gauge how healthy your internal system is. Believe it or not, there's even a scale. It's called the Bristol Stool Form Scale, describing a range of faeces – from ones that look like rabbit pellets to water. We're aiming for Scale 4, the perfect stool, which should look like a big, pale brown sausage, smooth and soft! I'm sorry to be so descriptive, but a perfect poo means a happy, healthy colon and that means better health!

uterus

Some women have much heavier periods when they're on a long detox. Clients have complained they've had the worst and longest period ever, and they're always amazed when I excitedly explain how good this is! It's another sign that the body is busy unloading toxins and that you'll feel better eventually.

It's worth noting that post-menopausal women have lost one of their major routes of elimination. So, for them, it's even more important to make sure the colon is working as well as possible.

kidneys

The kidneys are two bean-shaped organs, just 10 cm long and 5 cm wide, which process about 150 litres (over 250 pints) of fluid a day. Remarkably, only about 1.5 litres (about 2½ pints) of that fluid leave the body as urine, 96 per cent of which is water – water that needs replacing! The rest is urea (found in many facial skin treatments!) and salts. The kidneys' main job is to keep blood composition constant by filtering certain waste products out.

As I mentioned previously, we're aiming to produce straw-coloured wee, to confirm that we've replaced enough of the water we're losing as urine. During the 48-Hour Plan you may well be peeing more than usual and, again, this is a good sign that the kidneys are working efficiently and that the cells are letting go of those toxins (especially if you're weeing more than usual at night). Welcome this even if it's a bit inconvenient. You can make up for a disturbed night by resting during the day. Remember, this is your plan and your time to do whatever you want to do!

16.
The Plan!

Congratulations! You're now ready to do the 48-Hour Plan to a healthier life. Hopefully, by now, you'll have tried some of the techniques, excluded a few of the 'naughty but nice' foods, cut down on a few of the external toxins and are looking forward to a thoroughly relaxing weekend.

I'm going to outline the order that worked for me. But, please, do your own thing in any order you prefer. My timetable should give you ideas about what you might want to do and when, taking you from first thing in the morning to last thing at night. But start your detox break at any time of the day. Plan ahead what you want to do at particular times of the day. I've included here all the techniques I would use in my Plan, and repeated the methods so that you don't have to keep flicking backwards and forwards in the book. But feel free to refer to the previous chapters for alternatives.

Doing the detox from a Friday lunchtime to Monday lunchtime worked for me because it's easier to follow a plan like this over a weekend when you have less reason to feel guilty. And starting halfway through a Friday gives you a full afternoon to relax and pamper yourself by trying out some of the suggested treats to turn your Weekend into a real spa experience.

You'll find recipe ideas in the next chapter, corresponding

to the time of year you have chosen, so you can try out your culinary skills when you've nothing else to do because you've turned the outside world off!

switch them off!

No TV!	No Mobile Phone
No Radio	No Watch
No Telephone	No Laptop

Don't panic when you look at that list and wonder what on earth you're going to do with all that time. If you feel bored and it's pouring with rain, you can play games such as Scrabble, patience or anything you fancy that isn't too competitive. Or you can read that book you've always meant to read. Or write a diary of your experiences. You can even rent a video if you're really at your wits' end, as long as it's an *under*-stimulating movie such as a romantic comedy. And as long as you don't get sucked into watching the TV and getting back in touch with the world!

If at any point you do start feeling lousy, just take it easy and reread chapter 9 on immune responses and how to deal with them. Don't forget, this weekend isn't supposed to make you miserable – it's supposed to refresh you and make you feel as if you have had a week's break with added health benefits.

suzi's optimum plan

friday

Lunch

Post-lunch rest

Afternoon relaxation: reading, walking

Pampering session: facial, etc.

Supper

Post-supper rest

Relaxation exercises

Bath before bedtime

Early to bed

saturday

Wake up naturally.

Wash your face and eyes.

Have a drink and snack/liver flush.

Evacuation

Clean your tongue, teeth and nose.

Breathing exercises – *Pranayama*

Tibetan whirling

Yoga exercises

Skin-brushing and shower

Self-massage

Meditation

Breakfast

Exercise outdoors

Lunch

Repeat this routine over the three days of the Weekend. I'm leaving some space here for you to add other activities or techniques you want to try.

I also want to try:

friday lunch

Eat as early as you can. This is your most important meal of the day and the one you'll most successfully digest and burn off. Remember not to drink any water *with* your food. Have a glass of room-temperature water an hour before your lunch and wait another hour after lunch till you have the next glass. Eat slowly. If you want a relaxed digestion and an end to bloating (often caused by bolting your food down!) chew each mouthful at least 20–30 times.

after lunch rest

First of all, rest immediately after eating. If you're anything like me, this might be the first time in your life when you sit down and do absolutely nothing for a *minimum of 15 minutes after eating*! I can't emphasize this enough. Don't read, talk or start making lists of what you're going to do for the rest of the Weekend. Just sit and 'be' – your digestion will really appreciate it.

afternoon relaxation

Try relaxing activities all afternoon. Maybe go for a walk, read, sleep, or do all three! And pamper yourself with one of the spa treats.

personal pampering in your own home spa

This section is essential for learning to pamper yourself and look after all your senses. It's your reward for working so hard on your diet, techniques and exercise all weekend. Here are some suggestions to exercise two of your neglected senses at the same time – *smell and touch*!

1. FACIAL: CLEANSE AND EXFOLIATE

1 tablespoon oatmeal or crushed almonds
1 teaspoon grated orange peel
1 teaspoon lemon or lime juice
1 teaspoon clear honey
1–2 teaspoons olive or linseed oil

Blend all the ingredients together with your fingers in a small bowl. Massage the mixture into your skin, rubbing gently in a circular motion, and then rinse off with plenty of warm water. (Yum! The ingredients are as good for your insides as they are for your skin – you can always lick them off if you're suffering from food deprivation!)

2. FACIAL: STEAM

You can make your own facial steam by adding 2–3 drops of your favourite essential oils to a bowl of very hot water. Lean over the bowl, put a towel over your head, close your eyes and inhale. Spend 5 minutes allowing your pores to open.

OR

Fill a basin with hot water, add 2–3 drops of the essential oil, soak your flannel thoroughly, wring out the excess water and place it over your face to open up the pores. Repeat several times.

3. EASY MOISTURIZING MASK FOR FACE, HANDS AND FEET

2–4 tablespoons clear honey
2–6 teaspoons coconut milk
8–10 drops vitamin E oil
10 drops of your preferred essential oil
1 teaspoon lemon juice
1 large cucumber – remove the skin and thinly slice ¾ and
    set aside. Blend or liquidize the remaining ¼ cucumber
    to use in the mask

In a bowl, mix all the ingredients together (apart from the cucumber slices), till you're happy with the consistency. Pat the mixture on to your face, feet and/or hands. Massage in gently and then leave for 15–20 minutes. Remove the mixture with warm water. Then lie down and cover your whole face, hands and feet (if you can) with the cucumber slices. Cucumber is full of silicon and sulphur for strong skin, nails and hair – so you might want to try this mixture as a hair treat as well. Leave the slices on for 15 minutes and relax . . . relax . . . relax. Rinse off with cool water and pat dry. If you're using this mixture as a hair treatment, use cider vinegar for the final rinse.

Then moisturize your skin by using the oils you've already chosen and mixed for your massage.

4. SCRUBS FOR BODY, FEET AND HANDS

3–4 tablespoons olive oil
10 drops of your favourite essential oil
1–2 tablespoons sea salt or sesame seeds

Mix the essential oil with the olive oil in a bowl and then add the sea salt or sesame seeds. Rub the skin gently with the mixture from top to toe and concentrate on your feet and hands if you're giving yourself a manicure or pedicure afterwards. Shower off with warm water. Your skin should feel really soft and smooth.

5. PEDICURE AND MANICURE

There are various ways of getting your feet and hands ready. The benefits of mustard foot baths are legendary, so you might want to try this, or one of the other foot baths mentioned in chapter 8. Or you could soak your feet or hands in a bowl of warm water infused with a couple of drops of an essential oil. Whatever you choose, use the suggested body scrub as an exfoliator, the moisturizing face mask as a treatment, and finish off with an oil massage.

6. FACIAL MASSAGE

Warm a teaspoon of your mixed oils in your palms. Rub your hands together and then press them all over your face quickly and firmly. Using your fingertips, tap lightly and quickly all over your face, starting from the centre and working outwards: along your eyebrows, under eyes, along the cheekbones, around your mouth and along your chin. Then, using your fingers, make little circles starting at the hairline and working down round the outside of the face. As you reach the chin, gently pinch the flesh between fingers and thumbs, working from the point of the chin to the ears. Then using the index fingers and thumbs gently pinch the eyebrows, moving outwards. Massage the middle of your forehead and the temples in circular motions. With two or three of your middle fingers, start at the nose and gently sweep along the bone under the eye, moving *out* from the nose towards your ears. Do the same under the cheekbones, sweeping outwards from nose to ears. Then put your fingers under the middle of your nose and sweep downward above the mouth, following the line of your upper lip. And put your fingers under the middle of your bottom lip and sweep upwards and out, again following the line of your lip. Finish the face by pulling on the ear lobes and give them a good massage. This will help the blood flow to your face and wake up your complexion. Lastly, rub your hands together quite fast and then place them over your face, keeping your eyes closed. Inhale the essential oils and the heat radiating from your hands.

supper and post-supper rest

There are lots of ideas in the recipe section. Try to eat your last meal of the day around 6 p.m. And remember to rest for at least 15 minutes after eating. After this you might like to have a detoxifying bath or just relaaax . . .

evening relaxation exercises

Lie flat on your back with your feet apart, the toes rolling away from the heels. Your arms are at your sides and slightly away from the body, with the palms facing up. Make sure your head is straight and your neck is long. Allow your mind to help the body relax and repeat mentally to yourself as you travel through the body, beginning with your toes, 'I relax my toes . . . my toes are relaxed. I relax my feet and ankles . . . my feet and ankles are relaxed. I relax my legs . . . my legs are relaxed. I relax my hips . . . my tummy . . . my arms . . . my chest . . . my back . . . my neck . . . my face . . .' until you reach your head and finally your mind. *Relax. Relax. Relax.*

a bath before bedtime

You should be in just the right mood for a lovely soothing bath. Turn the bathroom into your very own sanctuary.

! TOP TIPS FOR SPA BATHS

Decorate the bathroom with crystals, pebbles or driftwood.
Turn the main lights off – use scented candles.
Use an essential oil burner.
Pop a few drops of essential oil into a small bowl of warm
    water and put it near the radiator.
Play soothing, relaxing music.
Put a couple of drops of your favourite oil on to a warm,
    damp flannel and put it on your forehead while you soak.
Fold up a small towel and put it behind your neck for
    support.
Use thick and fluffy towels to wrap yourself in when you
    come out.
Lie down and relax after your bath and have a glass of water
    or a herbal tea.

Choose either a bath with essential oils (use 3–10 drops of your favourite oil in a bath – or the same total number of drops of a combination of oils) – OR an Epsom salts bath.

EPSOM SALTS BATH

The temperature should be as hot as is comfortable. Add 1 cup (one 200 g packet) of Epsom salts to a full bath and soak in it for 10–20 minutes. Do this on the three evenings of the Plan. After the bath, wrap up warmly, drink plenty of water and rest.

> **WARNING: Do not have this bath if you have any circulatory or heart conditions.**

bedtime – early to bed

Try to get to bed by 10 p.m. Have some soothing music on in the background, read, or just lie there and meditate. Don't *try* and sleep, go with the flow. As long as you're resting, it doesn't matter if you don't fall asleep straight away.

wake up naturally on saturday morning

How early is up to your body! This should be the quietest time of the day for you – lie in bed and don't move for a while. Say thank you to the day, your god, yourself, whatever you believe in. Rub your hands together for a minute, then cup them over your face. This will help ground you. Stay there as long as you like.

wash your face and eyes

Splash your face with cool/cold water a few times. Massage your eyes by rubbing the eyelids gently. Blink your eyes half a dozen times and then rotate them in all directions: to the side, up, down, diagonally and then clockwise and anti-clockwise. This will help you feel more alert and fresh.

drink a glass of warm water with lemon juice and have a snack

Squeeze half a fresh lemon into a glass of warm or room-temperature water and drink up. This will really wake up your digestion. Have a snack of seeds, nuts and a piece of fruit if you're hungry. Chew very thoroughly.

or try the liver flush

Mix the juice of half a lemon, half a clove of garlic, crushed, a little grated fresh ginger and a dessertspoon of olive oil. Add a small glass of vegetable juice or vegetable stock, stir vigorously and drink.

evacuation

Sit on the loo and try to have a bowel movement – but don't strain. Don't worry if it doesn't happen. Use the time to do your breathing exercises or to sit and 'be'. If you want to help things along, raise your arms above your head. This opens up the colon and makes up for the fact that our bodies are in completely the wrong position to go to the loo. In cultures where people squat to go to the loo, colons tend to be far less sluggish. Raising your arms is almost as good as squatting!

clean your tongue, teeth and nose

To scrape the tongue, use a tongue scraper or a small spoon. Gently move from the back of the tongue forward until you have scraped the whole surface.

Then take a mouthful of warm sesame oil and swish it from side to side for 2–3 minutes. Don't swallow it. Spit out the oil, then massage your gums with your index finger.

Tap your teeth gently together 5 or 6 times. This should get that *prana* moving!

Put 3–5 drops of warm sesame oil into each nostril, to help clean the sinuses, and improve the voice, vision and mental clarity. (In arid climates or during cold winters when central heating dries the air, this will keep the nostrils lubricated. Some say the nose is the doorway to the brain – so give it a treat this Weekend.)

breathing exercises: *pranayama*

Sit comfortably with your spine as straight as possible.

Close your eyes and rest your left hand on your knee – you'll be using your right hand.

Keep your mouth shut throughout.

Using your right thumb, close off your right nostril. Then, through your left nostril, inhale slowly and deeply. Hold the breath for four counts.

Now with your middle fingers close your left nostril and exhale slowly out of your right nostril.

Then, keeping your left nostril closed, inhale through your right nostril, and hold the breath for four counts.

Move your thumb on to your right nostril and exhale through the left nostril.

Repeat the sequence using alternate nostrils for about 5 minutes.

tibetan whirling

Find a safe, big space. Stand up straight with your arms stretched out, parallel to the floor, and spin round clockwise until you become dizzy – it usually takes 5–6 times. Keep practising and adding revolutions as you get the hang of the technique. Make sure your feet are squarely on the ground throughout, and spin as fast as you can without falling over!

yoga exercises

If you're used to doing yoga, do as many sun salutations as you like. Six rounds would be good. Otherwise, choose your favourite asanas from below or try and do them all. You have the time now.

1. WARM-UPS

Use an old towel or a yoga mat to sit and lie on. Begin by lying down with feet apart; your toes should be rolling away from your heels, and your arms a little away from your body with the palms of your hands facing the ceiling. Close your eyes. Just allow the body to become quiet and still for about 2–3 minutes, releasing any tension you find, particularly in the hips, shoulders, chin and jawline. Have a really good, long stretch with your arms over your head.

Then come up to a comfortable sitting position on the floor, cross-legged, with your spine straight and your shoulders relaxed. Gently drop your head to your chest, stretching your neck. Take a few breaths and then gently turn your head twice to the right and twice to the left to ease any stiffness there. Don't take your neck back. Just roll your head from side to side a few times. Then interlock your fingers and stretch your arms out ahead of you, palms outwards. Take them up and over your head reaching as high as you can. Stretch the whole upper body to the left and then to the right, and release your arms. Then interlock your fingers behind your back and stretch your body forward as far as you can, keeping your head in line with your spine. Hold then release.

Then move on to some *leg lifts, which strengthen abdominal, back and leg muscles*. Lie on your back on the floor, arms by your sides and neck long (point the chin down towards your chest). Keep toes flexed towards your face. As you inhale extend the right heel and lift the right leg as high as you can. Keep the leg straight. Hold for a few breaths and then release on an exhalation. Repeat with the left leg. Alternate as many times as is comfortable. As one leg lifts the other one is also working by keeping itself strong along the floor with toes also flexed.

2. FORWARD BEND (*PASCHIMOTHANASANA*)

This is a seated posture, which is a complete stretch for the back of the body, massages all the abdominal organs and relieves constipation. It also counteracts obesity and strengthens and stretches the hamstrings (backs of thighs).

Sit with your legs straight out in front of you, with your toes flexed towards your face. Stretch your trunk upward, keeping the spine elongated, and raise your arms above the head as you inhale deeply. As you exhale, bend forward from the hips. Reach forward towards your feet and bring your chest down towards your thighs – only go as far as you feel comfortable. You are aiming towards your toes – take hold of your thighs, shins, or ankles – whatever you can reach. Hold as long as is comfortable, and then inhale and stretch your arms and body back up. Repeat several times for maximum benefit. Then lie down and rest your back.

3. LOCUST (*SALABHASANA*)

This is one of the back bends, which increase flexibility, rejuvenate the spinal nerves, and bring a rich blood supply to the vertebrae. This particular one also strengthens the lower back, abdomen, thighs, and hips, and stimulates the adrenal glands and kidneys.

Lie on your tummy with your legs together and your toes pointing away from the body. Place your arms at the sides of your body, with the palms down. As you inhale lift both legs up and pull your arms back and away from the body, raising your chest and arms off the floor. Hold for several breaths, then release. Repeat once or twice more. Then rest.

Follow this with two inverted postures – the most beneficial of all asanas, because the heart is higher than the head, increasing the supply of oxygen to the brain and allowing the heart to rest, as gravity helps to return de-oxygenated blood to it.

4. DOG HEAD DOWN (*ADHO MUKHA SVANASANA*)

This stretches the back, legs and ankles, and massages the abdominal muscles.

In a kneeling position place your hands on the floor so that they're immediately below the shoulders, just in front of you. On an exhalation, raise your hips into the air, lifting your knees off the floor, to form an inverted 'V'. Press your chest towards the floor, while lifting and pointing your tailbone upwards. Drop your head towards the floor. Lift as high as you can, and then release your heels towards the floor, giving a good stretch to the legs. Don't force your heels down. Keep your arms and legs as straight as you can. Hold for as long as is comfortable, and then release. Repeat.

5. HALF SHOULDERSTAND (*ARDHA SARVANGASANA*)

WARNING: This is potentially a very beneficial exercise, but do not attempt it if you've ever had any neck problems.

This one benefits the whole body. The thyroid gland is massaged together with the other endocrine glands: so it's fantastic for the immune and nervous systems, and brings peace and stillness to the mind.

Lie on your back. Using your arms for support, raise your legs and buttocks into the air, while keeping your legs together. Place your hands on your buttocks to support your back. Your arms will be at an angle from the body. Press your neck to the floor AND DO NOT, WHATEVER YOU DO, TURN YOUR HEAD TO THE RIGHT OR LEFT. This can be really dangerous. Try to hold the position for several minutes and when ready, roll each vertebra back to the floor, from the top of the spine to the bottom, keeping your head on the floor if possible. Extend your legs and rest for several minutes.

This should be followed by the Bridge as a counterpose to stretch your back out.

6. THE BRIDGE (*SETU BANDHASANA*)

This stretches and strengthens the neck and loosens the shoulders, and improves spinal flexibility.

Lie on your back with your knees bent, your heels close to your buttocks and your feet as far apart as your hips. With your arms at your sides, inhale and raise your hips, rolling each vertebra up until you're resting on your shoulders. Bring your hands on to the back with the fingers pointing towards the spine and the thumbs around the waist. Your feet, shoulders, neck, back of the head and upper arms are supporting your body. Feel the stretch in your thighs, back, neck and shoulders. Keep your knees, feet and legs parallel. Breathe deeply and hold as long as is comfortable. Release by slowly rolling down.

7. FINAL RELAXATION – THE CORPSE (*SAVASANA*)

Just as it's important to begin every asana session with a period of relaxation, it's also essential to finish with one of about 10 minutes. This gives the physical and mental energy released by the asanas an opportunity to circulate properly.

Lie flat on your back with your feet apart, and your toes rolling away from the heels. Have your arms at your sides and slightly away from your body, with the palms facing up. Make sure your head is straight and your neck is long. Allow your mind to help the body relax and repeat mentally to yourself as you travel through the body, beginning with your toes, 'I relax my toes . . . my toes are relaxed. I relax my feet and ankles . . . my feet and ankles are relaxed. I relax my legs . . .' and so on, until you reach your head and finally your mind. Relax. Relax. Relax. Stay there as long as you like, you might even fall asleep!

Allow your breathing to deepen and bring yourself back,

stretching your legs and arms and then rolling to the right –
stay there for a couple of minutes before coming up to a
comfortable cross-legged position. With your hands on your
knees, keep your eyes closed and spend a minute or two
following your breathing.

skin-brushing and shower

Before showering, on dry skin, start brushing firmly UP
TOWARDS THE HEART, starting from the soles of your
feet. Work up the front of each leg to your abdomen. Brush
your tummy with circular movements in a CLOCKWISE
direction. Carry on brushing upwards to the bottom of your
breasts. Then work all the way UP the back of your legs, past
your bottom, as far as you can reach, and brushing as vigorously
as feels comfortable. The bottom and thighs are good areas to
concentrate on as they usually carry the most fat cells!

When you get to your upper chest and upper back, change
the direction and start brushing from the neck DOWN-
WARDS TOWARDS THE HEART, both front and back,
always in the direction that the blood flows to the heart. Finally,
brush your hands and all the way UP each arm, on the top and
the underside. And don't forget to brush inside your armpit by
holding your arm up and brushing DOWNWARDS.

Don't do your face, but you can give the back of your
neck and your scalp a good going over!

Follow this with a shower and when you've reached the
end of your ablutions turn the shower on as cold as you can
stand it for 10 seconds (building up over the Weekend to 30
seconds), then turn it up to warm again for a minute or two.
Repeat this three or four times and end on cool.

Your skin should be pleasantly warm and damp after your shower. Use your choice of carrier and essential oils. Mix 3–6 drops of the essential oil with the carrier oil in a little bowl. Make sure you put plenty of the mixed oils on your hands or fingers, so that these glide over your skin easily.

Again, as with the skin-brushing, always work towards the heart, but this time start with the head. Sit on the edge of the bath, on the loo, or on a towel on the floor – whatever is comfortable.

HEAD

Begin by concentrating on your scalp, as this will help prevent any detoxing headaches and keep you calm. Sit up straight (with your back supported if possible). Slowly 'shampoo' your scalp all over, using the pads of your fingers, not your nails, working the oil well into the scalp. This movement is incredibly relaxing as well as being very good for your hair. Leave the oil on your scalp while you carry on with the rest of your massage.

You can repeat the face massage from Friday afternoon, or go straight to your neck and shoulders.

NECK AND SHOULDERS

Very hard to do on yourself, but what you can do, with a well-oiled hand, is to pinch the flesh along the top of your shoulder blade, between the first three fingers and thumb of the opposite hand, moving up and down the entire length of each shoulder. And then, with one hand, very gently massage the back of your neck.

ARMS

Try and cup the whole of the opposite arm by placing your fingers on top and your thumb underneath. Start at the wrist point and, using upward strokes, glide up the arm, pressing firmly. Repeat several times on each arm, alternating between thumb on top and thumb underneath.

FEET

In a seated position, put a foot on the opposite knee. Cradle your toes in the same-side hand, and with your opposite hand, using your knuckles only, circle all over the bottom of your foot. Squeeze the back and sides of the foot above the heel. This is where a lot of tension is held. Finish by pulling each toe firmly and briskly, making sure each one is oiled. Repeat on the other foot.

LEGS AND THIGHS

With one foot up on the side of the bath, cup your two hands around both sides of the leg, from above the anklebone, and firmly and slowly glide both hands together right up the leg and over the knee. You might have to do this several times to make sure your whole leg has been massaged. Re-oil your hands and repeat the same on your thighs as high up as you can, but this time you can use more pressure. Repeat on the other leg.

ABDOMEN AND BOTTOM

For the abdomen, just use circular movements, in a clockwise direction, as gently or as firmly as you feel comfortable with. A lot of people don't like having their tummies massaged so see how you feel. The bottom is a very difficult muscle to work on your own, so instead give it a good scrub with a loofah when you're next in the shower!

Don't wash the oils off – allow them to soak into your skin for added benefits.

meditation

With your shoes off, sit cross-legged on the floor or, if you have trouble keeping your spine straight, sit with your back against a wall. Or sit on a chair, as long as it's straight-backed and your feet are resting comfortably on the floor. (Or even lie down – I don't recommend this as I always fall asleep!) Sit with your palms up and open like empty bowls, resting on your knees.

Close your eyes. Keep them relaxed and imagine there is a white dot between your eyebrows. Breathe normally, but as you inhale and exhale, gradually begin to notice your breathing. Don't try and influence your breathing in any way, just follow it. Allow it to reach its own rhythm.

If your brain starts getting busy and making lists, don't try to stop it. Look at each thought, imagine it in a bubble and just blow it away. Then come back to following your breathing, and stillness.

At the end of the meditation, sit quietly and let your body come back to the present.

breakfast

This could be taken at any stage; you don't have to wait till you've completed all of the above suggestions. See the recipe section for ideas. Suzi's Smoothie should give you enough energy to go for a long walk, but there are other suggestions. Don't forget to rest for 10–15 minutes after eating, even if it's a 'liquid' breakfast.

exercise outdoors

You need to get that precious sunlight into your body, even if it's the middle of winter. Go for a brisk walk for as long as you like *but for a minimum of 30 minutes* to get everything moving. Try to walk fast enough to feel light sweat on your forehead and under your arms.

If you want to lose weight and ensure strong bones exercising is *essential*.

! TOP TIPS FOR WALKING DURING THE WEEKEND PLAN

Make sure you've first warmed up your muscles by doing some stretching (or yoga) exercises.
Keep your head and shoulders relaxed.
Wear loose comfortable clothes and good trainers or shoes.
Take a waterproof instead of an umbrella, to free yourself up.
Swing your arms to get your heart pumping even more.
Towards the end of your walk, slow down and cool down.
Stretch all the muscles you've been using and take your time, don't rush.

By the time you've done all of the above you'll be ready for lunch, so after this go back to the beginning of this chapter and start pampering yourself all over again. Be adventurous with the recipe suggestions in chapter 17, and try as many different ones as you can over the course of the Weekend. By Monday lunchtime you'll have completed 48 hours to a healthier life and, although you may feel a little rough on the first day, by the end you should be feeling rested – and ready for more! See chapter 18 for ideas on how to 'carry on in the real world'.

17. Recipe Suggestions

The Weekend diet should be composed of as much 'plant' food as possible: fresh fruit and vegetables, seeds and nuts, brown rice and pulses. And remember, of course, 2 litres of water a day! I've divided up the recipe suggestions into two sections – one for an autumn or winter detox; the other for a spring or summer cleanse.

reminders and guidelines for an eating plan over the weekend

Peel, top and tail any vegetables or fruit – especially if juicing and using non-organic produce.

Keep the water from steaming or cooking vegetables and use it as stock.

Do *not* fry in linseed oil. Stir-fry ingredients in a little water first and when the food is cooked, take the pan off the heat and *then* add the linseed oil. This stops the oil from oxidizing and is healthier. You may substitute olive oil for linseed oil, but use half the recommended amount (*cooking* with olive oil is allowed occasionally for baking vegetables or making soups).

A little peanut butter, soya or coconut milk may be used in

moderation in certain recipes, *but the emphasis is on moderation*!

Soak nuts, seeds and dried fruit overnight to make them more digestible. Or toast nuts and seeds in a wok/frying pan for one minute (with nothing added) to make them even tastier.

Tamari and black or cayenne pepper can all be used as seasoning – but, again, in moderation.

NOTE ON MEASUREMENTS

In order to simplify the recipes – and so that you don't have to worry about weighing everything out pedantically, or get stressed as to whether a rented-cottage kitchen is well equipped – I'm using a *cup* for larger measurements. This is the equivalent of about 250 ml – just under 9 fl oz (or just under $^1/_2$ pint), and should represent the volume of a standard coffee mug. (I'll be using cups for ingredients like rice, as well as liquids.)

autumn/winter

breakfast

Breakfast can be as light or filling as you like. Even in winter my breakfast smoothie keeps me going for hours. But if you need something a bit more substantial you can go for porridge with a little soya milk, or any other cereal, as long as it isn't made from wheat. There are plenty of millet, corn or quinoa alternatives on sale in health shops, but for maximum cleansing try to keep to a fruit, seed and nut only breakfast or the smoothie.

suzi's smoothie

(per person)

1 apple or pear
1 kiwi fruit
2–3 strawberries, and a few blackberries, blueberries or
**   raspberries – any berries including frozen ones**
1 teaspoon–1 tablespoon of lecithin granules
1–2 tablespoons of linseed oil
1 tablespoon of soaked golden linseeds, with the water
Handful of ground pumpkin & sunflower seeds
2–4 almonds and 1 brazil nut
Cranberry, apple or any fruit juice if you need more liquid
1 tablespoon of aloe vera juice (optional)

The linseeds should be soaked overnight.

Peel and chop up the fruit, as required. Put all the ingredients in a blender, and whizz up. Add fruit juice if the consistency of the smoothie isn't quite right. Add a little dried fruit (a date or two) if you really need to increase the sweetness.

lunch

Lunch should be your main meal of the day during a detox, and the earlier the better. And I can't think of anything better than steamed vegetables and brown rice when it comes to a cleansing meal – especially during the winter! In an ideal world, your evening meal should be a much lighter supper, such as vegetable soup (with a little brown rice added for bulk if necessary). There are sauce suggestions to jazz up the rice, and some alternatives if you really can't bear it for three days. But, hopefully, you'll at least *try* the steamed veg and brown rice.

So *how much* should you eat? You can choose any vegetables from the list and eat as much of them as you like. Within reason, you can also eat as much brown rice as you like. It's so good at cleaning your gut, I don't mind if you eat it all Weekend!

But, if you need a guideline on quantities, try to eat little and often – this is easier on the digestion than waiting till you're really ravenous and stuffing yourself silly. Make each meal no bigger than the amount of food it would take to fill (generously) your two hands, and you'll be helping your digestion even more. (And lucky you if you have huge hands!) If you want to eat four small brown-rice-and-steamed-vegetable meals a day, that's fine. But everyone has a different appetite, and I don't want you to go to bed hungry and miserable.

SUGGESTED VEGETABLES

These are the most nutritious ones, and they're well suited to steaming.

Broccoli	Swiss Chard
Brussels Sprouts	Green Beans
Cabbage	Mangetouts
Kale	Carrots
Cauliflower	Fennel
Spinach	Leeks
Bok Choy	Okra

brown rice

Of course there will be cooking instructions on the packet, but here are some tips to help you cook perfect brown rice.

RICE **TOP TIPS**

Don't wash the rice because it has already been cleaned and you may remove important nutrients (remember it contains an oil that helps heal the gut).

Measure the rice by volume not weight. Fill a standard coffee mug with rice and use double this amount of *cold* water. That should make enough rice for two of you, or for two meals if you're on your own. If you want to cook more than one meal's worth just double the quantities: two mugs of rice with four mugs of water.

Use a wide, shallow saucepan with a lid (I use my wok). Once the water has come to the boil, turn the heat down to the lowest possible setting. Leave the lid on and don't keep lifting it to peek, as this will lengthen the cooking time. Equally, don't stir the rice – the grains are delicate and if you stir them during cooking they break, releasing the starch inside and turning sticky.

Brown rice usually takes 40–45 minutes to cook. Then take it off the heat and leave the covered pan to stand for a further 5-10 minutes. Fluff up the rice just before serving.

If you've cooked extra rice for another meal, leave it to cool right down before putting it in the fridge. This could take up to an hour, depending on the quantity you've cooked.

The Food Standards Agency advises keeping cooked rice, in the fridge, for no longer than 24 hours but, by their own admission, they are erring on the side of caution because an extremely nasty tummy bug (called Bacillus cereus) can proliferate in warm cooked rice. My advice would be to cook enough for meals over 48 hours and keep the rice in a fridge, in a bowl covered with cling film or in a container with a lid, *for no longer than two days*. And make sure you heat it through very thoroughly if you're using it for a hot meal. (To reheat it, put the rice in a pan with a couple of tablespoons of water and warm through on a gentle heat, shaking the pan from time to time.) Whatever you do DON'T leave cooked rice out overnight in a warm kitchen.

You may find plain brown rice just too boring to have three days in a row, so here are some suggestions to liven it up.

stir-fried rice

(per person)

Small piece (to taste) fresh ginger, finely chopped
2–3 cloves garlic, finely chopped
1 cup cooked basmati brown rice
Few dashes of tamari (to taste)
1–2 tablespoons linseed oil

In a wok or large frying pan heat 2 tablespoons of water till it's simmering (preferably water the vegetables were cooked in). Add the ginger and garlic, then add the rice and stir very fast with a wooden spatula for a few minutes, until the rice is hot through. Add the tamari and oil once the pan is off the heat. (As I've already mentioned, this prevents the oil from oxidizing.)

You can add other herbs and spices that you enjoy to the cooking water.

If you need even more excitement, look at these suggestions, which complement brown rice and vegetables.

avocado sauce

(2 portions)

1–2 ripe avocados (1 big one or 2 small ones), peeled and
   diced
2 cloves fresh garlic, crushed
Juice of 1–2 lemons
Dash of Tabasco
Pinch of dried chilli
A little soya or rice milk (optional)

Put all the ingredients in the blender and whizz them up together. Serve the sauce with steamed vegetables and brown rice, either poured over these, or as a side dish. You can make the sauce runnier by adding a little soya or rice milk, or blend it briefly only so it's thick and chunky.

green sauce

(2 portions)

2 cloves garlic, chopped
Ginger (to taste), peeled and chopped
2–3 teaspoons rice vinegar (or cider vinegar)
1 cup chopped fresh coriander

¼ cup of water
2 tablespoons honey

Put all the ingredients into a blender, or use a hand liquidizer, and whizz up till you get a smooth paste. Again, this can be poured over the rice and vegetables.

healthy tomato sauce

(4 portions)

1 red onion, chopped
2 cups water/stock
½ teaspoon fresh red chillies, finely chopped and deseeded
2 teaspoons fresh oregano, off the stalks
4 cloves garlic, chopped
2 standard cans (2 × 400 g) chopped tomatoes (with juice)
Nori flakes or tamari as salt substitute and pepper (to taste)
Bunch fresh basil, coarsely chopped or torn
Linseed/olive oil to taste

Cook the chopped onion in a couple of tablespoons of the water or stock till it starts softening. Add the chillies, oregano and garlic. Simmer for 2 minutes, then add the chopped tomatoes and remaining water/stock. Leave to simmer for a further 30 minutes. Add salt flavouring (if required) and the fresh basil. Remove the pan from the heat and add a little oil to taste.

All you need to do for the next two sauces is pop all the ingredients into a blender, and whizz them up until you get the consistency you prefer.

sundried tomato sauce

(2 portions)

A small jar (250 g) sundried tomatoes, drained
2 cloves garlic, chopped
2 tablespoons linseed oil
Add any herbs you like. (I love this with fresh basil.)

spinach & basil pesto

(2 portions)

2 cloves garlic, chopped
Nori flakes or tamari and pepper to taste
¼ cup sunflower seeds
⅓ cup pine nuts
1 bunch fresh basil
2 cups fresh spinach
1–2 tablespoons linseed oil

The next three side dishes will make brown rice and vegetables a *protein-complete meal*, and a lot more exciting. Pulses such as chickpeas are needed to turn a carbohydrate-based meal – such as brown rice and vegetables – into a protein-rich meal. It won't hurt you to live *without* animal protein for three days. You'll be getting enough protein from the seeds and nuts you'll be snacking on between meals, and more than enough from the following dishes. If you intend to follow this plan for much longer than three days, it's definitely worth giving these suggestions a whirl.

tahini sauce (my favourite)

(per person)

1 tablespoon tahini paste (lightest and runniest you can find)
2 cloves garlic, crushed
Juice of 1–2 lemons
A little soya or rice milk (if needed)

Just whizz up in the blender and pour over the steamed vegetables and brown rice.

hummus

(2 portions)

1 standard can cooked chickpeas, drained
Juice of 1–2 lemons (to taste)
1–2 teaspoons tahini
2 cloves garlic, crushed
1–2 tablespoons olive or linseed oil
Parsley for decoration
Tamari and pepper (to taste)

Again, just put all the ingredients into the blender and whizz up. You can drizzle a little olive oil over the hummus once it's blended, and keep it in the fridge. This is a protein-packed side dish, which can be eaten with raw vegetables (and salads in summer) or served with hot rice and vegetables.

dhal

1 cup dried red lentils
Tamari (to taste)
1 teaspoon turmeric powder
2 fresh chillies, deseeded
1 tomato, chopped
1 tablespoon linseed oil
1 teaspoon cumin seeds
1 onion, finely sliced
2 cloves garlic, finely chopped
Fresh coriander (to taste)

Wash the lentils in a sieve in cold water until it runs clear. Put them in a pan and cover them with cold water to about 2 inches above the lentils. Bring the water to the boil – skim off the foam that appears. Then simmer the lentils until they become mushy; if they get too thick, add more water. Add tamari and half of the turmeric powder. Split the chillies into four and add these and the chopped tomato to the lentils. Meanwhile heat 1 tablespoon of water/stock in a separate pan. Put in the cumin seeds, remaining turmeric powder, onion and garlic and cook till soft. Then add all these to the dhal, plus the chopped coriander. Simmer on a low heat for 40–60 minutes, with the lid on. Add water if needed to prevent sticking. Add the linseed oil when the pan is off the heat.

You'll notice olive oil creeping into these recipes. You can't use linseed oil for *cooking*, so use olive oil instead for *roasting* vegetables, and for some of the soups. You can always add a little water (but NOT when the oil is already hot and on its own in the pan, as it will spit) to make it go further.

crispy broccoli

I'm including this recipe because it's yummy and broccoli is simply the best, nutritionally! You can try this with any other vegetables to spruce them up a bit.

(1–2 servings)

1–2 head broccoli, broken into florets
Olive oil
Nori flakes and pepper (to taste)
2 cloves garlic, finely chopped
2 pinches cayenne pepper
1 tablespoon sesame seeds

Just pop the broccoli florets into a baking tray, and drizzle the oil and sprinkle the spices and sesame seeds all over them. Bake on a medium heat till they've gone all crispy – usually for 10–20 minutes.

You can also do this with any vegetables you have left over after steaming them.

ROOT VEGETABLES

Carrots (top of the crops!)	Swede
Turnips	Celeriac
Parsnips	Sweet Potato

Root vegetables will be in season at this time of the year but they don't steam very successfully (apart from carrots) and need to be baked in lots of olive oil to be really interesting. They are also very high in starch and quite challenging for the digestion. However, in moderation, they are a good substitute, especially if you can't tolerate brown rice. Roots can either be baked as above, or boiled and mashed up with a little olive oil and flavourings.

suzi's mild vegetable curry

This is really a cross between a stew and soup and is a good one to make when you have loads of vegetables that you want to cook in one go. Perfect for a detox weekend!

The longer and slower the curry cooks the tastier it becomes (and especially if you leave it overnight to marinate). Use a nice big saucepan and just keep adding chopped vegetables till the pan's nearly full, making sure you add enough stock so that the veg is well covered by liquid. You can always add more stock and flavouring later, if it starts to look too thick.

(3–4 portions)

Broccoli, carrots, fennel, 1–2 sweet potatoes, okra, parsnips, leeks, kale – any mixture of vegetables you like, peeled and cubed.

Juice of 1 lime
1 mango, chopped into tiny pieces
Fresh coriander, chopped (to taste)
2 fresh red chillies, de-seeded and finely chopped
Ginger (to taste), finely chopped
2 teaspoons Garam Masala
2 cups (about 1 pint) vegetable stock (or more!)
2 tablespoons either coconut milk or almond flakes. (Add to taste.)

In a jug, mix the lime juice, mango, spices and herbs together and set to one side. Make enough vegetable stock (from left-over cooking water or from a vegetable stock cube) to cover all the cubed vegetables in a large saucepan. Add the mixture of juice, spices and herbs, and stir through. Simmer on a very low heat, with the lid on, for about an hour. After that, if possible, leave it sitting on the stove (with the heat off) till needed to give all the spices and herbs further time to seep into the vegetables. Heat the curry up, add the coconut milk or almond flakes at the last minute, and serve with cooked basmati brown rice. You might like to sprinkle sesame seeds over the stew to add a little protein.

thai sauce

If you don't like Indian food, you can make a stew very similar to the above curry (and which will also see you through the Weekend) using Thai spices instead. Again, cook any combination of vegetables you like in at least 1 pint (2 mugs) of stock to make sure they're well covered, adding this sauce.

1 onion, finely chopped
1–2 cloves garlic, finely chopped
Galangal (a lovely sweet ginger) (to taste)
1 stick lemon grass, finely chopped
3–4 fresh lime leaves
Sweet basil (to taste)
1–2 fresh red chillies, deseeded and finely chopped
1 tablespoon coconut milk

Put all the ingredients in the blender and whizz them up. If necessary, add more coconut or soya milk to make the sauce runnier. The sauce will keep in the fridge to use later. This is so much nicer than any of the shop-bought ready-made Thai sauces and the spices are all good detoxifiers! It's quite strong, so add to your stew to taste.

soups for supper

red pepper soup

(2 portions)

1 red onion, chopped
3 cloves garlic, finely chopped
1 medium sweet potato, peeled and cubed
2 teaspoons paprika
½ teaspoon chilli powder or 1 teaspoon cayenne pepper
2 tablespoons chopped fresh coriander
2 cups shredded cabbage
2 cans tinned tomatoes (with juice)
5 cups vegetable stock
1 tablespoon honey
1–2 fresh red chillies, deseeded and diced

2 tablespoons olive oil
2 red peppers, deseeded and diced
½ cup coconut milk
Tamari and pepper (to taste)

Cook the onion, garlic, sweet potato, all the spices (apart from the chillies) and seasoning in a couple of tablespoons of water for 5 minutes. Add the cabbage, tomatoes, vegetable stock, honey and chillies. Simmer until the potato is cooked. Take off the heat and add 1 tablespoon of olive oil. In another saucepan, sauté the peppers in the remaining oil (*just this once!*) till soft. Add the peppers to the soup, plus the coconut milk and any more seasoning. Purée when cool. Serve hot with polenta slices – just delicious.

carrot and coriander soup

(2 portions)

1 large red onion, chopped
1–2 tablespoons olive oil
3 cloves garlic, crushed
2 tablespoons fresh marjoram or 1 teaspoon dried
3 tablespoons chopped fresh coriander (set a couple of
  stalks aside as garnish)
6 large carrots, peeled and diced
1 sweet potato, peeled and diced
4 cups vegetable stock
Cayenne pepper and tamari to taste

Fry the onion in 1 tablespoon of olive oil for 5 minutes, then add the garlic, marjoram and chopped coriander and cook for a further minute. Then add the carrots and sweet potato and sauté for a minute or two. Transfer everything to a big saucepan. Add the vegetable stock to the pot and bring to the boil. Simmer until the carrots and the sweet potato are soft. Add seasoning to taste. Purée when cool. Reheat and garnish with coriander to serve.

healthy vegetable soup

(1–2 portions)

You can also make a filling and warming soup by first dissolving an organic vegetable stock cube in 2 cups (1 pint) of boiling water and, once the cube is dissolved, adding the stock to a saucepan containing any combination of chopped-up vegetables you fancy. Add garlic, herbs and seasoning and leave to simmer on a very low heat for an hour or so, making sure the vegetables are well covered by the liquid. You'll notice there is *no oil* used in this soup, which makes it a little less tasty but much more cleansing! If you want to bulk the soup up, add a handful of pulses, such as lentils or chickpeas, and a handful of brown basmati rice. This would make a complete protein and carbohydrate meal.

alternatives to rice

MILLET

Millet, as you've seen in chapter 5, is the king of the grains when it comes to detoxing. Millet usually needs more water to cook in than rice – 3 cups of water to 1 cup of millet – but check the instructions on the packet. You can add millet to soups and stews or cook it on its own to eat with one of the side dishes as a cleansing alternative to rice. To improve its texture and make it tastier, you might like to toast it in a little oil before cooking.

millet with squash

(4 servings)
½ **red onion, chopped**
2 **carrots, peeled and diced**
1 **head broccoli, diced**
¼ **medium squash or pumpkin, peeled and cubed**
2 **cups millet**
6 **cups water**
Seasoning to taste
Toasted sesame seeds

Put all the vegetables at the bottom of a large saucepan. Add the millet, water and seasoning. Cover the pan and bring to the boil. Simmer for 30 minutes. Stir through and serve with tahini sauce or sprinkled with toasted sesame seeds.

QUINOA

Quinoa doubles in size when it's cooked, so you don't need to start off with much of it.

quinoa and vegetable sauce

(1–2 servings)
½ **cup quinoa**
1 **cup water**
1 **tablespoon olive oil**
1 **red onion, finely chopped**

½ bunch fresh coriander, chopped
1 fresh red chilli, deseeded and chopped
Any vegetables you fancy, chopped finely. Peppers are good
    for this dish.
1 standard can chopped tomatoes, with juice

Place the quinoa in a pan with the water and bring to the boil. Simmer on low for 10–15 minutes, then strain the quinoa and set it aside. Meanwhile, in another pan fry the onion in the olive oil until it's soft, then add the coriander and chilli. After a further minute, add all the vegetables, cover and sweat for 5–10 minutes. Then add the chopped tomatoes and cook for another 10 minutes. Try to time it so that the quinoa's ready at the right moment, or warm it gently through. Serve with the vegetables on top.

POLENTA

Now this *is* a really tasty alternative to brown rice and, as it's made from corn, is entirely suitable for use during the Weekend.

polenta with olives and sun-dried tomatoes

(2 servings)
4 cups soya milk
1 tablespoon olive oil
Tamari (to taste)
1½ cups polenta
10 black olives, stoned and finely chopped
6 sun-dried tomatoes, drained and finely chopped
1 bunch fresh basil, finely chopped

Combine the soya milk, olive oil and tamari in a big saucepan. Bring this to the boil, reduce the heat to low and then slowly pour in the polenta, whisking it constantly. After 3 minutes, add the chopped-up olives, sun-dried tomatoes and most of the basil. Stir for another minute, then take the pan off the heat. The mash should be creamy in texture, like porridge. If it isn't, add more soya milk or water.

Transfer the polenta into a baking tray and smooth it out using the back of a spoon. Leave it to cool for a few hours. It hardens up to a quiche-type consistency and you'll then easily be able to cut it into pieces. Heat it up by popping slices under the grill. It's delicious as a snack and with soups (or served with a big salad in summer). Garnish it with basil leaves.

puddings

I haven't mentioned puddings because there aren't any really healthy substitutes for home-made apple pie or fudge ice cream! We're trying to break the need for sweet things this Weekend, but if you're really miserable and craving a pudding, snack on dried fruit and nuts – in moderation. As a winter dessert, pop a couple of pears or apples on to a tray and bake them until soft in the oven. Drizzle honey over them once they are cooked. Add some seeds, and you have a wonderfully healthy and warming winter pud!

spring/summer

You should be able to make raw fruit, vegetables, juices and cold soups the mainstay of your Plan at this time of year. There are also suggestions on more filling meals if you need them.

Brown rice is still important for its cleansing properties so, even if you only use it in a salad, make sure you eat sufficient amounts of it throughout the Weekend, as well as nuts, seeds and pulses.

breakfast

Again, you can start the day with a handful of nuts, seeds and fruit or Suzi's Smoothie. You may want to kick off the day with a juice as well.

juices

If you have a juicer, you can juice almost any fruit or vegetable you like. If you don't have one, don't panic – *fruits* will benefit you almost as much if they are liquidized or blended. But you can't really successfully liquidize or blend *raw vegetables*. So if you're keen to have juice-only meals this Weekend make sure you add a teaspoon of spirulina or freeze-dried wheat grass to your fruit blend to make up for the lack of green vegetables. (These 'wonder foods' are available at most health shops.)

SUZI'S 3 FAVOURITE JUICES

For these suggestions you *will* obviously need a *juicer*. Raw vegetables liquidized in a blender just won't taste as nice. (However, if you *don't* have a juicer and *really* want to try these, you can always chop the vegetables up into very, very small pieces, and make sure the juice is sweet enough by adding more chopped apple or a little honey. You may also need to add more water if it's too thick to drink.)

If you *are* using a juicer, you don't need to peel your fruit and veg and can even include the rind and pith of the lemon.

(But if you're using a blender, make sure you've peeled, cored and diced all the ingredients.)

Quantities are per person.

detoxifier

4 carrots
¼ large cucumber
1 cup spinach leaves
1–2 teaspoons aloe vera juice
OR:
4 carrots
1 apple
1 head broccoli
1 stalk fennel
2 sticks celery
Fresh ginger to taste
A little lemon to taste

liver supporter

This is a mixture of the 'liver *flush*' and a juice that will help *support* the liver.

½ raw beetroot (peeled)
2 sticks celery
2 apples
4 carrots
¼ lemon (including the rind and pith)
½ grapefruit
Fresh ginger to taste
Pinch cayenne pepper

(Don't worry if after drinking this juice you notice your wee or poos are a bit red – it's the effect of the beetroot, and it's quite normal!)

afternoon pick-me-up

4 slices pineapple
½ cup filtered water
½ cucumber
2 red apples
1 heaped teaspoon spirulina or wheatgrass
Fresh ginger to taste

summer soups

gazpacho

(2 servings)
1 small red onion, finely chopped
3–4 tomatoes, peeled and deseeded
1 red pepper, deseeded
1 cucumber
1–2 tablespoons brown rice vinegar (or cider vinegar)
3–4 tablespoons olive or linseed oil
2 cloves garlic
½ carton tomato juice
Tamari and pepper to taste
2 spring onions, finely chopped
Fresh parsley and basil, marjoram or thyme

Purée or blend the chopped onion, tomatoes, half the red pepper, and half the cucumber and transfer to a large bowl. Add the vinegar, olive oil, garlic, tomato juice, and seasoning to taste. Finely chop the spring onions, the rest of the cucumber and red pepper and fresh herbs and sprinkle over the soup. Refrigerate for two hours. Delicious and cooling in the summer and quite filling. Add sunflower or sesame seeds instead of croutons!

spinach and avocado chilled soup

(2 servings)

1 large packet (500 g) fresh spinach
2 cups soya milk
2 cups vegetable stock
2 big ripe avocados
Dash of Tabasco
Juice of 2 limes
Tamari and pepper to taste
Parsley for garnish

Chop the stalks off the spinach, wash the leaves and place them in a pan with 2 tablespoons of water. Cover the pan and cook on a medium heat for 5 minutes. Add the soya milk and stock. Bring to the boil, cover the pan and simmer for 10 minutes, stirring occasionally. Leave to cool, then purée and pour into a bowl. Peel and stone the avocados and purée them with a little of the soup. Stir this into the rest of the soup. Cover the bowl with cling film and chill in the fridge for 2 hours. Before serving, add the Tabasco and lime juice, and any seasoning required, and garnish with parsley.

cleansing watercress soup

(2 servings)

3 cups vegetable stock
3–4 spring onions, finely chopped
Mixed fresh herbs, chopped
1 sweet potato, peeled and sliced
2 bunches watercress, chopped
½ cup soya milk
Lemon or lime juice to taste
Tamari and pepper to taste

Heat one cup of stock in a large pan. Add the spring onions and herbs, cover and simmer for 5 minutes. Add the sweet potato and the rest of the stock to the saucepan, cover and simmer for another 20 minutes, or till the potato is cooked. Add the watercress to the pan and simmer for a further two minutes. Take the pan off the heat and add the soya milk. Stir well and leave till cool. Then blend the soup until smooth and creamy. Reheat, and add the lemon or lime juice and seasoning to taste before serving. Or refrigerate for two hours to serve chilled.

cooked veg dishes

vegetable skewers with thai satay sauce

Allow enough vegetables to fill 2 skewers per person.
Cut into cubes aubergines, courgettes, mushrooms, artichoke hearts, peppers, onions and tomatoes — any

combination you fancy. Put them on skewers, brush them with olive oil and pop the skewers under the grill for a few minutes on each side.

For the *Thai satay sauce*, mix 2 teaspoons of peanut butter (as organic and salt-free as possible!) with 1 teaspoon of the Thai sauce in the Winter section, and up to a tablespoon of water or soya milk to thin it, if needed. Either pour this over the hot skewers, or dip the cubes into it, one by one! Serve with a portion of brown rice for extra bulk.

colourful baked vegetables

(2 servings)

1 red pepper

1 yellow pepper

1 orange pepper

1 aubergine

2 courgettes

1 large red onion

4 tomatoes

3 cloves garlic, crushed

Tamari and pepper to taste

1–2 tablespoons olive oil

Juice of 1 lemon, or 1 tablespoon brown rice vinegar (or cider vinegar)

Deseed the peppers and slice them into quarters. Cut the aubergine, courgettes, onion and tomatoes into small chunks and put them all in a baking tin. Sprinkle plenty of crushed garlic, tamari and pepper and pour a little olive oil all over them, and bake at a low to medium heat till cooked and slightly brown – usually about 45 minutes. You may need to add a little more oil to stop the veg from burning. Once cooked, dress the vegetables with lemon juice or brown rice vinegar and a little more olive oil. Leave them to cool in the pan in the marinade. Serve with basmati brown rice and a dollop of hummus or tahini sauce on top.

salads

First of all, here are a couple of dressings that should make you enjoy even more those lovely and healthy summer salads.

cheat's mayo

I can't tell you how delicious this is and there isn't a trace of an egg in it. If you're missing your mayonnaise or creamy dressing and are going to eat a lot of salads over the Weekend, try this. Make sure you only use *silken* tofu or it's quite revolting!

1 teaspoon capers
2 large cloves garlic, crushed
2 tablespoons lemon juice
½ teaspoon French mustard
1 tablespoon brown rice vinegar (or cider vinegar)
Tamari to taste
1–2 tablespoons olive or linseed oil
10 oz silken tofu (usually ½ large packet)
(Soya milk or water to thin mixture if necessary)

Just combine all the ingredients in a blender and adjust the quantities for taste and texture.

french dressing

2 teaspoons brown rice vinegar (or cider vinegar)
Dash lemon juice
½ teaspoon honey
Pinch mustard powder
1 clove garlic, crushed
Tamari to taste
3–4 tablespoons olive or linseed oil

Put all the ingredients in a screw-top glass jar (put the lid back on!) and shake vigorously. You can keep the jar in the fridge for the Weekend – just give it a good shake before using it.

a medley of raw vegetables

Make up a platter of raw carrot batons, broccoli florets, green beans, sliced peppers – anything you fancy! – and serve it with hummus or any other side dish, plus one of the suggested dressings.

suzi's summer salad

This is *my* favourite summer salad.

(2 servings)
1 packet mixed salad leaves
1 bunch watercress
1 carrot, peeled and grated
½ green pepper, deseeded and sliced
1 ripe avocado, sliced

4 spring onions, finely chopped
2 sundried tomatoes, finely chopped

Combine the mixed salad leaves, watercress and carrot in a large dish. Arrange the pepper and avocado on top of these. Sprinkle over the spring onions and sundried tomatoes. Add your favourite dressing.

suzi's summer salad #2

(2 servings)

1 small packet fine green beans
1 head broccoli, chopped into florets
2 large carrots, peeled and thinly sliced
1 stalk fennel, finely sliced
1 small cooked beetroot, peeled and finely sliced
½ cucumber, finely sliced
1 packet mixed salad leaves
2 spring onions, chopped

Steam the green beans and broccoli and leave to cool. Arrange the finely sliced carrots, fennel, beetroot and cucumber on a bed of salad leaves. Sprinkle the chopped spring onions and drizzle one of the suggested dressings all over. Add slices of avocado and some sesame seeds or pine nuts to make this salad more substantial. You can also substitute any other green vegetables you love for the beans and broccoli.

aduki bean salad with avocado sauce

(2 side portions)

1 standard tin (410 g, 220 g drained) cooked aduki beans, drained and rinsed
½ cucumber, finely chopped
2 tomatoes, finely chopped
1 stick celery, finely chopped
1 spring onion, finely chopped
Fresh basil and chives to taste
Avocado sauce (as explained in Winter section)

Mix all the ingredients together in a bowl, and add the avocado dressing.

mixed pulses salad

(2 side portions)

1 standard tin cooked mixed beans
1 small red onion, finely chopped
1 tablespoon chopped fresh parsley

Combine the ingredients in a bowl and add a dressing to make a tasty and cleansing side salad.

quinoa salad

(2 servings)

1 cup quinoa
2 cups water
1 red onion
1 red pepper
½ cucumber
3 tomatoes
1 tablespoon chopped chives
1 tablespoon chopped parsley
1 tablespoon chopped mint
French dressing

Rinse the quinoa well and strain. Put it into a saucepan with 2 cups of water. Bring this to the boil, then simmer, covered, for 10–15 minutes. Then take the pan off the heat and leave it to cool. Strain if necessary. Peel the vegetables and dice them into tiny cubes. Mix these and the herbs into the cooled quinoa in a salad bowl and drizzle the dressing over.

brown rice and shitake mushroom salad

(2 servings)

1 red onion, chopped
1 punnet shitake mushrooms, sliced
2 big tomatoes, diced
½ cucumber, diced
1 tablespoon chopped fresh parsley
2 spring onions, chopped
1 cup cooked brown rice

Sauté the onion in a little olive oil, till golden and soft. Then add the mushrooms and sauté till cooked. Leave them to cool, before combining all the ingredients in a bowl and adding dressing.

puddings

If you're really missing your pud and need something sweet, you can have a little 'live' yogurt with honey, or chopped fruit, or seeds and nuts. Or all of them combined, which would make your pudding almost a meal in itself!

18. How to Carry on in the Real World

The Weekend is over and you're either dying to get back to eating and drinking 'normally' or have decided to go for an optimum cleanse of three to six weeks! (The longer you follow the Plan, the better you'll feel and the longer you'll *want* to follow it.) Either way, well done for making it so far and I hope you've acquired new skills for looking after your own well-being and your family's health for ever.

For those who want to continue with a wheat- and dairy-free diet there are a few more meal suggestions that include fish, soya products and goat's cheese. You'll find these dishes much easier to incorporate into your life. This is still a fairly cleansing diet – but a little more acidic. If you don't want to follow any more diets, at least now you know which foods are packed with nutrients and which aren't.

And you know which lifestyle changes have made you feel better and which haven't. Whatever you decide to do for the rest of your life, try and look after *you* by incorporating some of the techniques mentioned previously and in this chapter. See how you can integrate at least 10 minutes of 'me' space into your busy day. Learn how to make time to develop all your senses and pamper yourself a bit more. See how to get regular exercise, no matter what, and how you can lead a more toxin-free life.

carrying on – the essentials:

Further diet suggestions

Exercise

Cutting down on outside toxins

Integration

Sensism

further diet suggestions: quick and easy wheat- and dairy-free meals

These meal and snack suggestions are designed for people who have no time to prepare homemade soups and bowls of brown rice on a daily basis but want to stick to a healthy eating plan. If you do want to continue with the cleanse, it will be easier to spend a quiet Sunday preparing some of your meals for the week ahead and store them in the refrigerator or freezer (but my smoothie will NOT keep).

breakfast

Suzi's Smoothie

Or add linseeds, linseed oil and lecithin to a shop-bought smoothie.

Organic millet flakes with goat, soya or rice milk

Organic wheat-free muesli with goat, soya or rice milk

Porridge

Fruit salad (or stewed fruit in the winter)

A handful of nuts and seeds and a piece of fruit

Organic free-range egg and wheat-free toast

Goat's cheese on wheat-free toast

lunches

Prepare these at home and take them in to work.

Smoothie

Hummus with carrot batons and other raw veg or salad

Roasted vegetables, brown rice and tahini paste

Homemade vegetable soup

Avocado sandwiches (Mash avocado with lemon juice, pepper, garlic and a little olive oil. Use wheat-free bread.)

Sandwiches with wheat-free bread and tuna, mackerel, salmon or chicken

lunch – if you can't take food into work

Your choice will obviously depend on what's available at your work canteen or the shops and cafés near your workplace.

Try a salad bar – have lots of the vegetables and whatever else you can trust.

Takeaway sushi – most supermarkets and some fast-food chains sell it now.

Takeaway salad with hummus or goat's cheese

Takeaway vegetable soup

Oily fish such as salmon or mackerel with salad or vegetables

Baked potato with coleslaw or baked beans

snacks

Pumpkin, sunflower & sesame seeds

Unsalted nuts

Dried figs, apricots & dates

Raisins

Fresh fruit

Baked Salmon Cover the fish with fresh herbs, such as dill or tarragon, add a little white wine and bake in foil. There is no need to add oil; the salmon has enough of its own! Serve with steamed vegetables such as broccoli or spinach. If you want more bulk or have a hungry partner, also serve basmati brown rice or a baked potato, with a little butter.

Stir-Fry Try a stir-fry with soya sausages, as they are surprisingly tasty. Cut up any carrots, broccoli and greens you have, or use a packet of prepared stir-fry vegetables. Add some soya sausages, chopped up into small pieces. Fry the healthy way – using stock or water initially, and adding oil at the end off the heat. Use flavourings such as tamari and garlic or a spoonful of tahini paste. You can also add a drop of white wine, some tomato purée, anything that will give even more flavour to the dish – as long as it's chemical-free.

Goat's Cheese Grilled on Wheat-Free Toast with added relish such as seaweed tartar (available in a good organic shop) or organic chutney. This can be served with a rocket side salad and vinaigrette dressing.

Tinned Sardines on Wheat-Free Toast

Whitebait with Wheat-Free Toast

Organic, Sugar-Free Baked Beans on Toast

Wheat-Free Pasta with a tomato sauce and a big green salad.

OILS

For optimum EFA consumption, you might like to continue – whenever possible – cooking your food without oil and drizzling linseed oil over the meal once it's off the heat. Failing that, you can use olive oil in the same way. And if you need olive oil for baking, add a tablespoon of water for every tablespoon of oil. You'll use less oil and your food shouldn't stick to the pan.

PUDDINGS

Try *Soya or Tofu* puddings, ranging from yogurts to cheese-cake, which are on sale in health stores and some supermarkets. And there's always *fresh fruit*, of course!

! TOP TIPS FOR EATING HEALTHILY

Once a week have a 'no solids' day.

Make breakfast and supper light meals – eat your main meal at lunchtime.

Leave 4 hours between meals.

Eat in the quiet and always sitting down.

Don't talk while chewing and chew each mouthful at least 20 times.

Eat slowly, put cutlery down between each mouthful.

Exercise your taste buds by blocking your nose.

Eat till comfortably full, not stuffed.

Don't drink water *with* your meals – drink 30 minutes to 1 hour before eating and wait 1 hour after eating.

Avoid ice-cold food and drinks.

Concentrate on eating alkaline foods.

exercise

You don't need me to remind you how important exercise is for the rest of your life. Decide what you enjoy and make sure you find enough time to do it – NO MATTER WHAT – your health, heart and bones depend on it!

> 30 minutes, 5 days a week – that's only 2.2% of the total waking week. You *do* have the time. It's just habit to think you haven't.

Remember these?

! TOP TIPS FOR BUILDING UP TO 30-MINUTE WALKS

Get off the bus or train one stop earlier and walk the rest.
Walk at lunchtime.
Walk the children to and from school – it will benefit their health too.
If you play golf, walk as fast as possible between holes.
Use the stairs instead of the lift, and walk up escalators.
Park your car in the bay furthest away from the supermarket entrance.
Walk to the local shops & use a rucksack to even out the load.
Don't use the TV remote!
Take longer walks at the weekend.

cutting down on outside toxins

I, for one, haven't managed to cut down on computer and TV use very much, but I *have* got rid of the electric blanket and clock-radio from my bedroom! We can't live without our electrical gadgets, but for the sake of our long-term health and our over-stimulated senses, we should at least question *how* we use them.

> **! TOP TIPS** FOR USING ELECTRICAL APPLIANCES
>
> Keep electrical appliances at least 1 m (3 ft) from the bedhead.
>
> Sit at least 1 m away from the TV.
>
> Use the laptop off the batteries whenever possible.
>
> Sit at arm's length from the computer screen.
>
> Don't use a hair dryer after 7 p.m. The EMFs could interfere with melatonin production and disrupt your night's sleep.
>
> Give your wristwatch a holiday at weekends or during leisure time.
>
> Keep calls short on cordless and mobile phones.
>
> Set your washing machine to run at night.

air purifiers!

And if all else fails, here is a list of plants that have been rated as being the best for removing indoor toxins. They're especially good at absorbing chemical emissions from computers, and can also improve the moisture content of a dry work or home environment.

Ivy	Potted Gerbera
Palms	Dracaena, e.g. Dragon Tree
Boston Fern	Rubber Plant
Weeping Fig	Potted Chrysanthemum
Peace Lily	Spider Plant

So fill your home or office with plants!

integration

Finding time every morning to do yoga and go through the nose-clearing and tongue-cleaning techniques can be a tall order. I have a very quick routine to ensure that body, mind and spirit are all catered for each and every day – no matter what. Just 10 minutes in the morning and at night is all it takes. *When I have more time, I do more!* Again, it's up to you to choose the techniques and exercises you really enjoy and that you can easily incorporate into your own routine.

morning routine

Quiet time in bed for 2–3 minutes
Warm water and lemon drink
Tibetan whirling
Tongue-scraping/teeth cleaning/nose clearing
Pranayama breathing while sitting on the loo!
Skin-brushing
Hot & cold shower
Quick facial massage using daily moisturizer – not oils

Quick DIY massage – using body lotion rather than oils – on legs and arms only

Quick walk for 10 minutes or yoga exercises

evening routine

Yoga exercises, gym session or a long walk for 30 minutes–1 hour

5–10 minute meditation

sensism

Finally we need to consider our five senses. Experimental Psychologist Dr Charles Spence believes there is a new philosophy, which he has called *sensism*, that we need to embrace if we are to increase our well-being.

According to Dr Spence, the senses are so intertwined that most people can't tell the difference between an apple and an onion if they eat them with their nose pinched shut. In order to get the senses more balanced and integrated we therefore need to stimulate them regularly – a sort of sensory workout!

hearing

Search out natural sounds, such as running water, rustling leaves, birdsong. Make a point of 'listening' to natural sounds whenever you can (and turn the mobile off so you're not disturbed). Listen to beautiful music that inspires and relaxes you. Background music has a profound effect on how we feel and act – just ask the supermarket giants!

sight

Get out into the sunlight as much as possible – even if only for five minutes at a time – during the day. Think about colours for your home and clothes that might affect your mood, such as energizing reds and calming blues and greens. Get plenty of colour into your food as well: red, orange and yellow foods are full of antioxidants.

taste

Incorporate these six tastes into your daily diet so your taste buds get as much exercise as your body: *sweet* (dates), *sour* (yogurt), *salty* (tamari), *pungent* (ginger), *bitter* (leafy greens) and *astringent* (pulses).

smell

If possible, have an essential oil burner sitting on your desk. According to Dr Spence, the smell of lavender oil balances and stimulates office workers and can make them more productive and efficient. It can even change their voices so they *sound* more relaxed! And 80 per cent of a food's flavour comes from its smell, so close your eyes and take in your meal's aromas next time you sit down to eat.

touch

This is the most neglected of the five main senses, according to Dr Spence's research. He believes we crave touch and that having massages will address this, as well as relieving stress and tension. What more of an excuse do you need to make sure you get a regular massage? And before you say you can't possibly afford it, just check out your local colleges. Massage courses need guinea pigs for students to practise on. This usually means extremely cheap, but effective, massages!

Dr Spence also suggests that we surround ourselves with tactile, natural objects, such as pebbles or driftwood, to feel and touch: 'The irregularities of natural objects are probably more attractive to us because irregular shapes were all we touched thousands of years ago, before we evolved.'

. . . and not forgetting the sixth sense

This is the one we women recognize and rely on more than all the others: *intuition*. It will be very well looked after if you practise a little meditation or relaxation each day – even if only for five minutes. Anything that stills the mind, even if you just sit in silence and stare at the walls, is going to help the development of your sixth sense.

Your intuition will, I hope, keep you and your family on the road to a Healthier Life. It's your body and if you stop for long enough to listen to it, it will tell you everything you need to know! Whatever you decide, make it work for you. I know how easy it is to feel you don't have one spare minute in a day. So you may decide to dedicate only 50 per cent of your life to optimum health. It doesn't matter, as long as *some* of the healthy habits stay with you.

If you want to cleanse for only one day a week, that's fine. If you eat meat and two veg every Sunday lunchtime, that's fine too – just make it meat and *five* veg from now on! Whatever eating plan you follow, at least make sure that you *minimize* the 3 'S's – salt, sugar and stimulants – and *maximize* the EFAs by eating plenty of oily fish and drinking a daily smoothie that incorporates them all. *And drink 2 litres of water a day!* As I said at the beginning of the book, if you do no more than this you will be improving your long-term health more than you can possibly imagine!

Think about changing the proportions of healthy to unhealthy foods and practices in your diet and life rather than permanently going without things and feeling miserable. Life shouldn't be a battle, full of deprivation – it should be varied and full of fun. Remember:

90% optimum nutrition + 10% of what you fancy = perfect health!

I hope you've discovered how to balance your life so that your body, mind and spirit *and* all your senses feel healthier, and continue to do so, long after the Weekend is over. And if the stress and toxins start to build up again, just take another 48 hours out and revisit the road to a healthier life. It will always be there for you – you have the map now.

Good luck and good health!

acknowledgements

A huge thank you to all the experts who willingly backed up my beliefs with their sound, scientifically based quotes; to Louise Moore, Saskia Janssen, Elisabeth Merriman and everyone else at Penguin for their fantastic support, encouragement and editorial improvements; to Janie Hildebrand and Patricia Haygarth for their contributions; to Barbara Wren of the College of Natural Nutrition for inspiring me in the first place; and to my agent Ruth Katz without whom I wouldn't have got this far! Finally, a big thank you to Cathy McClure, David Collett, Jill Brett, Martyn Levett, Emma Green, Ruth and Micky, and all my friends and family, whose belief in me got me through the tough days!

further reading and information

READING

F. Batmanghelidj, MD, *Your Body's Many Cries for Water* (Global Health Solutions)

Tony Buzan, *The Mind Map Book* (BBC)

Udo Erasmus, *Fats that Heal, Fats that Kill* (Alive Books)

Elson M. Haas, MD, *Staying Healthy with Nutrition* (Celestial Arts)

Johanna Paungger and Thomas Poppe, *Moon Time* (The C. W. Daniel Company Limited)

Dr Charles Spence, *The Secrets of the Senses*, www.ici.com

ORGANIZATIONS

Allergy UK: www.allergyuk.org tel.: 020 8303 8583

Backcare: www.backcare.org.uk tel.: 020 8977 5474

British Association for Nutritional Therapy: www.bant.org.uk

The College of Natural Nutrition: www.natnut.co.uk tel.: 01884 252 703

Consensus Action on Salt and Health: www.hyp.ac.uk/cash tel.: 020 8725 2409

Electromagnetic Hazard and Therapy: www.em-hazard-therapy.com
    tel.: 0906 401 0237 (premium rates)

Natural Mineral Information Service: www.naturalmineralwater.org

Powerwatch: www.powerwatch.org.uk

Research Centre for Neuroendocrinology: www.bris.ac.uk/Depts/URCN

Soil Association: www.soilassociation.org tel.: 0117 929 0661

SUPPLIERS

For yoga mats, videos and books: agoy, www.agoy.co.uk tel.: 020 8933 8421

For the more unusual supplements/products mentioned in the book (e.g. castor oil and linseed oil), plus all vitamins and minerals: Nutri Gold, www.nutrigold.co.uk tel.: 01884 251 777